Peripheral Neuropathy Diet Cookbook

A Complete Guide with Healthy and Delicious Nerve Pain Relief Recipes to Managing Pain and Restore Normal Health with 21 Day Meal Plan

Maria Carter

Copyright© 2024 by Maria Carter

All rights reserved worldwide.

No part of this book may be reproduced or transmitted in any form or by any means, electronic or mechanical, including photo- copying, recording or by any information storage and retrieval system, without written permission from the publisher, except for the inclusion of brief quotations in a review.

Warning-Disclaimer

The purpose of this book is to educate and entertain. The author or publisher does not guarantee that anyone following the techniques, suggestions, tips, ideas, or strategies will become successful. The author and publisher shall have either liability or responsibility to anyone with respect to any loss or damage caused, or alleged to be caused, directly or indirectly by the information contained in this book.

Table of Contents

INTRODUCTION 6
   What is Peripheral Neuropathy? 7
   Causes and Symptoms of Peripheral Neuropathy... 7
   Health Benefits of Maintaining a Peripheral Neuropathy Diet 9

BREAKFAST RECIPES 11
   Quinoa Porridge with Berries and Almonds 11
   Spinach and Mushroom Scramble with Avocado 12
   Chia Seed Pudding with Blueberries 13
   Oatmeal with Walnuts and Flaxseeds... 14
   Sweet Potato and Kale Hash 15
   Veggie-Packed Omelette with Herbs... 16
   Coconut Yogurt Parfait with Mixed Berries.. 17
   Almond Butter Toast with Banana and Hemp Seeds 18
   Avocado and Tomato Breakfast Sandwich on Whole Grain Bread 19
   Turmeric-spiced oatmeal with Chia Seeds 20
   Buckwheat Pancakes with Fresh Berries 21
   Poached Eggs on a Bed of Sautéed Greens.. 22
   Banana and Almond Smoothie Bowl 23
   Millet Porridge with Dried Fruit and Pumpkin Seeds 24
   Sweet Potato Breakfast Bowl with Spinach and Tahini 25

LUNCH RECIPES 26
   Grilled Salmon Salad with Avocado and Lemon Dressing.. 26
   Quinoa and Roasted Vegetable Bowl 27
   Lentil and Spinach Soup 28
   Turkey and Veggie Lettuce Wraps 29
   Chickpea and Cucumber Salad with Tahini Dressing 30
   Baked Cod with Sautéed Greens and Garlic.. 31
   Veggie-Loaded Quinoa Stuffed Peppers 32
   Zucchini Noodles with Pesto and Grilled Chicken 33
   Curried Cauliflower and Chickpea Stew 34
   Wild Rice and Black Bean Salad with Citrus Dressing... 35
   Grilled Chicken and Mango Salad with Cilantro Lime Dressing.............................. 36
   Roasted Beet and Feta Salad with Walnuts 37
   Brown Rice Sushi Rolls with Avocado and Cucumber 38
   Mediterranean Chickpea and Farro Salad 39
   Spinach and Quinoa Wrap with Hummus... 40

DINNER RECIPES.. 41
   Baked Salmon with Roasted Brussels sprouts 41
   Grilled Chicken Breast with Sweet Potato Mash 42
   Turmeric-Ginger Chicken Stir-Fry with Vegetables 43
   Lentil and Vegetable Shepherd's Pie 44
   Quinoa-Stuffed Bell Peppers with Black Beans 45
   Baked Cod with Lemon and Garlic Green Beans... 46
   Grilled Tofu and Veggie Skewers with Brown Rice 47
   Chickpea and Spinach Curry with Cauliflower Rice 48
   Turkey Meatballs with Zucchini Noodles and Tomato Sauce................................... 49

Lemon-garlic shrimp with Roasted Asparagus 50
Moroccan-spiced vegetable Tagine with Couscous 52
Herb-Roasted Chicken with Root Vegetables 53
Grilled Eggplant with Chickpea Salad 54
Seared Tuna with a Quinoa and Kale Salad 56
Spaghetti Squash with Pesto and Roasted Vegetables 57
Baked Tilapia with Sautéed Spinach and Mushrooms 58
Black Bean and Sweet Potato Enchiladas 59
Black Bean and Sweet Potato Enchiladas 60
Roasted Turkey Breast with Mashed Cauliflower 62
Tempeh Stir-Fry with Broccoli and Peppers 63

SMOOTHIES AND DRINKS **64**

Blueberry-Spinach Smoothie with Chia Seeds 64
Almond Butter Banana Smoothie 65
Pineapple and Kale Anti-Inflammatory Smoothie 66
Turmeric Latte with Almond Milk 67
Strawberry and Avocado Smoothie 68
Green Tea and Ginger Elixir 69
Mixed Berry and Flaxseed Smoothie 70
Carrot and Ginger Juice with Lemon 71
Coconut Water with Fresh Berries and Mint 72
Orange-Turmeric Smoothie with Chia Seeds 73

SNACKS AND APPETIZERS **74**

Roasted Chickpeas with Paprika 74
Veggie Sticks with Hummus 75
Avocado-Stuffed Cucumber Boats 76
Almond-Coconut Energy Bites 77
Sweet Potato Chips with Guacamole 78
Baked Zucchini Fries with Spicy Yogurt Dip 79
Greek Yogurt with Walnuts and Honey 80
Kale Chips with Nutritional Yeast 81
Apple Slices with Almond Butter and Cinnamon 82
Baked Beet Chips with Tahini Dip 83
Edamame with Sea Salt and Lemon 84
Sliced Veggies with Sunflower Seed Pâté 85
Baked Carrot Fries with Curry Dip 86
Cucumber and Radish Salad with Lemon Vinaigrette 87
Mini Stuffed Bell Peppers with Hummus 88

SIDES AND SALADS **89**

Roasted Brussels sprouts with Balsamic Glaze 89
Quinoa and Cucumber Salad with Lemon Dressing 90
Sautéed Kale with Garlic and Lemon 91
Grilled Asparagus with Lemon Zest 92
Roasted Sweet Potatoes with Cinnamon and Olive Oil 93
Wild Rice Pilaf with Cranberries and Almonds 94
Cabbage Slaw with Apple and Carrot 95
Spinach Salad with Strawberries and Pecans 96
Mediterranean Couscous Salad with Feta 97
Broccoli and Almond Salad with a Honey Dressing 98
Roasted Carrots with Thyme and Olive Oil 99

Avocado and Tomato Salad with Balsamic Drizzle 100
Cauliflower Mash with Garlic and Olive Oil 101
Lentil Salad with Feta and Herbs 102
Grilled Zucchini with Lemon and Parmesan 103

DESSERTS **104**

Coconut Chia Pudding with Fresh Mango 104
Baked Apple with Cinnamon and Walnuts 105
Dark Chocolate Avocado Mousse 106
Blueberry-Almond Crumble 107
Baked Pears with Honey and Almonds 108
Chia Seed Pudding with Coconut and Berries 109
Banana Oat Cookies with Dark Chocolate Chips 110
Almond Flour Brownies with Walnuts 111
Pumpkin Spice Energy Balls 112

21 DAYS MEAL PLAN **113**

INTRODUCTION

Living with peripheral neuropathy can be difficult. Constant tingling, numbness, or burning sensations in your hands, feet, and other places can disrupt your everyday life. What if you could use food to help you manage these symptoms, minimize discomfort, and enhance your general well-being?

Welcome to the Peripheral Neuropathy Diet Cookbook! If you've picked up this book, you or a loved one may suffer from peripheral neuropathy, a nerve disorder that causes pain, tingling, or numbness in the hands and feet. Living with these symptoms can be difficult, but the good news is that eating the appropriate foods can help manage them and improve your overall health.

This cookbook is designed to make your trip easier and more delightful. The recipes on these pages are healthy and full of taste, color, and basic ingredients that make every meal enjoyable. This book focuses on healthy nutrients proven to improve nerve function, reduce inflammation, and promote overall balance. It empowers you to take charge of your health one meal at a time.

Whether you are just diagnosed or have been dealing with peripheral neuropathy for years, this book is intended to be both accessible and soothing. Each recipe is designed to be simple, even for people with hectic schedules or little culinary expertise. We've concentrated on ingredients high in vitamins, antioxidants, and healthy fats while avoiding highly processed meals that might cause inflammation.

From substantial breakfasts to nutritious lunches, fulfilling dinners, and delightful snacks, you'll find meals that are simple to prepare and high in nutrients that promote nerve function. More significantly, this book is about rediscovering the joys of cooking and realizing that every bite you consume has the potential to change your mood.

We hope this cookbook becomes a reliable partner in your kitchen, making the journey to improved health easier and more delightful. Let's go on this delectable adventure to control your symptoms, increase your energy, and live healthier.

What is Peripheral Neuropathy?

Peripheral neuropathy is a condition that affects the peripheral nervous system, which comprises all nerves other than the brain and spinal cord. These nerves connect the brain and spinal cord to the rest of the body, facilitating movement, sensation, and bodily activities such as digestion. When these nerves are injured, it can cause various symptoms depending on which ones are impacted.

Common symptoms of peripheral neuropathy include tingling, numbness, burning, and pain in the hands and feet. Some people may also notice muscular weakness, balance issues, or sensitivity to touch. It can impair the digestive system, blood circulation, and other vital bodily systems in more severe situations.

Diabetes, infections, accidents, certain drugs, and vitamin shortages are all potential causes of peripheral neuropathy. It can sometimes develop for no apparent reason. Managing this illness frequently entails addressing the underlying cause, if identified, and implementing lifestyle modifications such as eating a good diet, exercising regularly, and collaborating closely with healthcare specialists to alleviate symptoms.

Causes and Symptoms of Peripheral Neuropathy

Causes of Peripheral Neuropathy:

Peripheral neuropathy can develop for various reasons, and identifying the potential causes is critical for managing the illness. Listed below are some of the most prevalent causes:

Diabetes is a primary cause of peripheral neuropathy, particularly when blood sugar levels are not adequately managed. High blood sugar levels can eventually damage nerves, particularly in the legs and feet.

Infections: Lyme disease, shingles, and HIV can all damage nerves and cause peripheral neuropathy.

Injury or Trauma: Physical injury or trauma to the nerves, such as those sustained in automobile accidents, falls, or operations, can cause nerve damage.

Vitamin Deficiencies: A deficiency in critical vitamins, notably B vitamins (B1, B6, and B12), vitamin E, and niacin, can induce nerve injury and result in peripheral neuropathy.

Alcoholism: Chronic alcohol drinking can cause nutritional deficits and toxic effects on the nerves, resulting in neuropathy.

Autoimmune Diseases: Lupus, rheumatoid arthritis, and Guillain-Barre syndrome can cause the immune system to target nerves, resulting in nerve damage.

Toxins and medications: Toxins, such as heavy metals and some compounds, can cause nerve damage. Some medicines, particularly chemotherapy treatments, can produce neuropathy.

Inherited Disorders: Some people are born with hereditary diseases, such as Charcot-Marie-Tooth disease, which can progress to peripheral neuropathy over time.

Kidney and Liver Disease: When the kidneys or liver do not work correctly, waste materials accumulate in the blood, causing nerve damage.

Unknown Causes (idiopathic): Idiopathic neuropathy is a condition in which the reason for peripheral neuropathy remains unknown.

Symptoms of Peripheral Neuropathy:

The symptoms of peripheral neuropathy vary according to the nerves involved. It can impact the sensory, motor, and autonomic nervous systems. The following are some of the most prevalent symptoms:

Tingling or Numbness: People may have a "pins and needles" feeling or numbness in their hands or feet, which can spread to their legs or arms.

Scorching or Sharp Pain: Many persons with peripheral neuropathy experience scorching, sharp pain, or stabbing sensations in their afflicted locations.

Muscle Weakness: Damage to motor neurons can cause muscular weakness, making it difficult to move, grasp items, or do daily duties.

Touch Sensitivity: Some patients with peripheral neuropathy experience discomfort even with gentle touches. This is known as allodynia, a condition in which typical stimuli produce discomfort.

Loss of Balance and Coordination: Nerve injury in the feet or legs can cause falls or difficulties walking.

Changes in Skin, Hair, or Nails: Peripheral neuropathy can cause changes in the look of the skin, hair, and nails, particularly in the legs and feet.

Digestive Issues: Autonomic nerve injury can influence the digestive tract, resulting in symptoms such as constipation, diarrhoea, bloating, and difficulty swallowing.

Dizziness or lightheadedness. Autonomic nerve damage can impair blood pressure control, resulting in dizziness or fainting when rising abruptly.

Heat Intolerance: Some persons with peripheral neuropathy may have difficulties controlling their body temperature, resulting in heat intolerance or excessive perspiration.

Health Benefits of Maintaining a Peripheral Neuropathy Diet

Maintaining a peripheral neuropathy-specific diet can dramatically enhance your quality of life and help control the condition's symptoms. A well-balanced, nutrient-dense diet can improve nerve function, decrease inflammation, and boost overall well-being. Here are the main health advantages of adopting a peripheral neuropathy-friendly diet:

1. Promotes nerve health: A diet high in vital vitamins, particularly B vitamins (B1, B6, and B12), helps to preserve and repair nerves. These vitamins are essential for safeguarding nervous system function and avoiding future nerve damage, especially for those with peripheral neuropathy.

2. Reduces inflammation: Peripheral neuropathy can be made worse by inflammation. Anti-inflammatory foods like leafy greens, berries, almonds, and omega-3-rich seafood can help decrease inflammation. This can help with pain, tingling, and other symptoms linked with nerve injury.

3. Improves blood sugar control: Diabetes, one of the most prevalent causes of peripheral neuropathy, necessitates careful blood sugar management. A diet rich in whole grains, veggies, and lean meats can help control blood sugar. By controlling blood sugar levels, you can avoid additional nerve damage and limit the course of neuropathy.

4. Increases antioxidant intake: Antioxidant-rich foods, including fruits, vegetables, and nuts, help protect neurons from oxidative stress, which can lead to nerve damage. Antioxidants neutralize toxic free radicals in the body, lowering the risk of future nerve damage and promoting the body's ability to repair.

5. Improves circulation: Proper blood circulation is necessary to give oxygen and nutrients to the nerves. Certain foods, such as garlic, ginger, and citrus fruits, encourage increased blood flow, which can enhance nerve function and alleviate symptoms of peripheral neuropathy.

6. Increases muscle strength: Peripheral neuropathy can cause muscular weakness. A diet high in proteins, vitamins, and minerals promotes muscular health and prevents additional muscle atrophy. Fish, chicken, beans, and legumes are good sources of lean protein, which helps to keep muscles strong and functioning properly.

7. Lowers pain and nerve sensitivity: Certain minerals, such as magnesium and alpha-lipoic acid, found in spinach, broccoli, and almonds, have been demonstrated to help relieve nerve discomfort and sensitivity. Including these items in your diet may help to alleviate the pain caused by peripheral neuropathy.

8. Maintains a Healthy Weight: Extra weight can put a strain on your nerves, exacerbating the symptoms of peripheral neuropathy. A well-balanced diet rich in whole, unprocessed foods will help you maintain a healthy weight, reducing stress on your nerves and promoting general nerve health.

9. Boosts the immune system: A strong immune system is essential for those with peripheral neuropathy, especially if the illness is associated with autoimmune disorders. A diet high in fruits, vegetables, and whole grains boosts your immune system, allowing your body to fight against infections and inflammation that can exacerbate neuropathy symptoms.

10. Offers long-term symptom management: Sticking to a peripheral neuropathy-friendly diet can help control symptoms in the long term. Individuals may report less nerve discomfort over time, better blood sugar management (for diabetics), and improved general nerve function. Following this diet can improve your daily comfort and quality of life.

BREAKFAST RECIPES

Quinoa Porridge with Berries and Almonds

Prep Time: 10 minutes

Cook Time: 20 minutes

Serve: 2 servings

Ingredients:

- 1/2 cup of quinoa, rinsed
- 1 cup of unsweetened almond milk
- 1/2 cup of water
- 1/2 tsp cinnamon
- 1/4 tsp vanilla extract
- 1 tbsp maple syrup or honey (optional)
- 1/2 cup of mixed fresh berries
- 2 tbsp sliced almonds
- 1 tbsp chia seeds (optional)
- A pinch of sea salt

Instructions:

1. Mix the rinsed quinoa, almond milk, water, and a sprinkle of sea salt in a medium saucepan. Bring to a boil, then lower to a low heat and simmer for 15-20 minutes, or until the quinoa is tender and the liquid has been absorbed.
2. Combine the cinnamon, vanilla essence, and maple syrup or honey (if using). Mix well and simmer for 2-3 minutes to fully mix the flavors.
3. Divide the quinoa porridge into bowls, then top with fresh mixed berries, sliced almonds, and chia seeds (if using).
4. Serve warm, and enjoy a nutritious breakfast.

Nutrition Information (per serving):

Calories: 240 Protein: 8g Carbohydrates: 35g Fiber: 7g Fat: 8g

Spinach and Mushroom Scramble with Avocado

Prep Time: 10 minutes

Cook Time: 10 minutes

Serve: 2 servings

Ingredients:

- 4 large eggs
- 1/2 cup of mushrooms, sliced
- 1 cup of fresh spinach, chopped
- 1/2 small onion, diced
- 1 clove garlic, minced
- 1 tbsp olive oil
- 1 ripe avocado, sliced
- Salt and pepper, to taste
- A pinch of red pepper flakes (optional)
- 1 tbsp fresh parsley, chopped (optional)

Instructions:

1. Heat the olive oil in a medium pan over medium heat. Sauté the diced onion and garlic for 2-3 minutes, until the onion is tender and transparent.
2. Cook for another 3-4 minutes, until the mushrooms have released their moisture and turned golden brown.
3. Add the chopped spinach and simmer for 1-2 minutes or until wilted.
4. Mix the eggs, salt, and pepper in a small bowl. Pour the eggs into the skillet with the veggies and gently scramble until they reach the desired consistency.
5. Divide the scramble into dishes and top with fresh avocado slices. To enhance flavor, sprinkle with red pepper flakes and, if desired, parsley.
6. Serve warm and enjoy.

Nutrition Information (per serving):

Calories: 290 Protein: 12g Carbohydrates: 9g Fiber: 5g Sugars: 2g Fat: 24g

Chia Seed Pudding with Blueberries

Prep Time: 5 minutes

Cook Time: 4 hours (chilling time)

Serve: 2 servings

Ingredients:

- 1/4 cup of chia seeds
- 1 cup of unsweetened almond milk (or any plant-based milk)
- 1/2 tsp vanilla extract
- 1 tbsp maple syrup or honey (optional)
- 1/2 cup of fresh blueberries
- 1 tbsp sliced almonds (optional for topping)

Instructions:

1. In a medium dish or jar, combine the chia seeds, almond milk, vanilla extract, and maple syrup or honey (if desired).
2. Stir thoroughly to ensure that the chia seeds are uniformly dispersed. Allow it to settle for about 5 minutes before stirring again to avoid clumping.
3. Cover the dish or jar and refrigerate for at least 4 hours or overnight. The chia seeds will absorb the liquid, resulting in a thick pudding-like consistency.
4. After the pudding has set, divide it into dishes and garnish with fresh blueberries and sliced almonds, if preferred.
5. Serve cold, and enjoy.

Nutrition Information (per serving):

Calories: 180 Protein: 5g Carbohydrates: 17g Fiber: 10g Sugars: 6g Fat: 10g

Oatmeal with Walnuts and Flaxseeds

Prep Time: 5 minutes

Cook Time: 10 minutes

Serve: 2 servings

Ingredients:

- 1 cup of rolled oats
- 2 cups of water or unsweetened almond milk
- 1/4 cup of walnuts, chopped
- 1 tbsp ground flaxseeds
- 1 tbsp honey or maple syrup (optional)
- 1/2 tsp cinnamon
- 1/4 tsp vanilla extract
- A pinch of sea salt
- Fresh fruit (such as sliced bananas or berries) for topping (optional)

Instructions:

1. Heat the water or almond milk in a medium saucepan until it boils. Add a pinch of sea salt and toss in the oats.
2. Reduce the heat to low and simmer the oats for 5-7 minutes, stirring periodically, until the oats are cooked and the mixture has thickened.
3. Remove the pot from the heat and add the cinnamon, vanilla extract, and honey or maple syrup (if using).
4. Divide the oats into a bowl and top with chopped walnuts, ground flaxseeds, and fresh fruit.
5. Serve warm and enjoy.

Nutrition Information (per serving):

Calories: 280 Protein: 8g Carbohydrates: 38g Fiber: 8g Sugars: 6g Fat: 12g

Sweet Potato and Kale Hash

Prep Time: 10 minutes

Cook Time: 20 minutes

Serve: 2 servings

Ingredients:

- 2 medium sweet potatoes, peeled and diced
- 1 cup of kale, chopped (stems removed)
- 1 small onion, diced
- 1 red bell pepper, diced
- 2 cloves garlic, minced
- 2 tbsp olive oil
- 1/2 tsp smoked paprika
- 1/4 tsp ground black pepper
- Salt, to taste
- 2 eggs (optional, for serving)
- Fresh parsley, chopped (optional, for garnish)

Instructions:

1. Heat 1 tbsp olive oil in a large pan over medium heat. Cook the diced sweet potatoes for 10-12 minutes, stirring regularly, until softened and golden brown.
2. Combine the remaining tbsp of olive oil, the onion, red bell pepper, and garlic in the skillet. Cook for 5-7 minutes until the veggies are soft.
3. Combine the chopped kale, smoked paprika, black pepper, and salt. Simmer for 3-4 minutes or until the kale has wilted and everything is thoroughly mixed.
4. If using eggs, prepare them separately to your taste (scrambled, fried, or poached) before serving on top of the hash.
5. Garnish with fresh parsley and serve warm.

Nutrition Information (per serving, without eggs):

Calories: 280 Protein: 4g Carbohydrates: 38g Fiber: 8g Sugars: 10g Fat: 12g

Veggie-Packed Omelette with Herbs

Prep Time: 10 minutes **Cook Time:** 10 minutes **Serve:** 2 servings

Ingredients:

- 4 large eggs (or egg substitute for plant-based option)
- 1/4 cup of bell peppers, diced (any color)
- 1/4 cup of zucchini, diced
- 1/4 cup of mushrooms, sliced
- 1/4 cup of spinach, chopped
- 1 small tomato, diced
- 1 tbsp fresh parsley, chopped
- 1 tbsp fresh chives, chopped
- 1 tbsp olive oil
- Salt and pepper, to taste
- A pinch of red pepper flakes (optional)

Instructions:

1. In a medium bowl, mix the eggs with a touch of salt and pepper. Set aside.
2. Heat 1/2 tbsp olive oil in a medium pan over medium heat. Sauté the chopped bell peppers, zucchini, and mushrooms for 3-4 minutes, until softened.
3. Add the chopped spinach and diced tomato, and simmer for another 1-2 minutes, or until the spinach wilts and the tomatoes soften.
4. Remove the vegetables from the skillet and put aside. Wipe out the skillet and heat the remaining olive oil over medium-low heat.
5. Pour the whisked eggs into the skillet and let them cook for approximately 2 minutes or until the edges start to firm. A spatula gently raises the edges, allowing raw egg to ooze below.
6. Once the eggs have mostly set, spread the sautéed veggies over one side of the omelet. Sprinkle chopped parsley and chives over top.
7. Fold the omelet in half and cook for another 1-2 minutes until the eggs are thoroughly cooked.
8. Serve warm, sprinkled with red pepper flakes for added heat.

Nutrition Information (per serving):

Calories: 220 Protein: 12g Carbohydrates: 8g Fiber: 2g Sugars: 3g Fat: 16g

Coconut Yogurt Parfait with Mixed Berries

Prep Time: 5 minutes

Cook Time: None

Serve: 2 servings

Ingredients:

- 1 cup of coconut yogurt
- 1/2 cup of mixed fresh berries
- 2 tbsp chia seeds
- 2 tbsp unsweetened shredded coconut
- 2 tbsp granola (optional, for crunch)
- 1 tbsp honey or maple syrup
- Fresh mint leaves

Instructions:

1. At the bottom, place half the coconut yoghurt in two serving glasses or bowls.
2. Place a layer of mixed berries on top of the yogurt.
3. Add 1 tbsp chia seeds and 1 tbsp shredded coconut to the fruit.
4. Add another layer of coconut yogurt, then additional mixed berries.
5. If desired, sprinkle with oats for crunch and drizzle with honey or maple syrup for flavor.
6. Garnish with fresh mint leaves if desired, and serve immediately.

Nutrition Information (per serving):

Calories: 220 Protein: 5g Carbohydrates: 25g Fiber: 8g Sugars: 10g Fat: 12g

Almond Butter Toast with Banana and Hemp Seeds

Prep Time: 5 minutes

Cook Time: None

Serve: 1 serving

Ingredients:

- 1 slice whole grain or gluten-free bread, toasted
- 2 tbsp almond butter (unsweetened)
- 1/2 banana, sliced
- 1 tsp hemp seeds
- A pinch of cinnamon (optional)

Instructions:

1. Toast a slice of whole wheat or gluten-free bread until brown and crunchy.
2. Spread the almond butter evenly on the toasted bread.
3. Top with banana slices, putting them equally on the bread. Sprinkle with hemp seeds and cinnamon, if preferred.
4. Serve immediately and enjoy.

Nutrition Information (per serving):

Calories: 280 Protein: 8g Carbohydrates: 28g Fiber: 6g Sugars: 7g Fat: 16g

Avocado and Tomato Breakfast Sandwich on Whole Grain Bread

Prep Time: 5 minutes

Cook Time: None

Serve: 1 serving

Ingredients:

- 2 slices whole grain bread, toasted
- 1/2 ripe avocado, mashed
- 1 small tomato, sliced
- 1/4 tsp lemon juice
- Salt and pepper, to taste
- A pinch of red pepper flakes (optional)
- Fresh basil or spinach leaves (optional, for extra greens)

Instructions:

1. Toast the whole grain bread until golden and crisp. In a small bowl, combine the avocado, lemon juice, salt, and pepper to taste.
2. Spread the mashed avocado equally on two slices of toasted bread.
3. Put the tomato slices on top of one slice of bread. If you want a little kick, add some red pepper flakes.
4. For added taste and nutrition, layer fresh basil or spinach leaves on the tomato slices.
5. Close the sandwich with the second slice of bread and serve right away.

Nutrition Information (per serving):

Calories: 300 Protein: 7g Carbohydrates: 36g Fiber: 10g Sugars: 4g Fat: 17g

Turmeric-spiced oatmeal with Chia Seeds

Prep Time: 5 minutes

Cook Time: 10 minutes

Serve: 2 servings

Ingredients:

- 1 cup of rolled oats
- 2 cups of unsweetened almond milk (or water)
- 1/2 tsp ground turmeric
- 1/4 tsp ground cinnamon
- 1/4 tsp ground ginger
- 1 tbsp chia seeds
- 1 tbsp honey or maple syrup (optional)
- A pinch of sea salt
- Fresh fruit (such as sliced bananas or berries) for topping (optional)

Instructions:

1. In a medium saucepan, heat the almond milk (or water) to a boil. Add a pinch of sea salt and toss in the oats.
2. Reduce the heat to low and simmer for 5-7 minutes, stirring regularly, until the oats soften.
3. Mix in the turmeric, cinnamon, and ground ginger. Continue heating for another 2-3 minutes or until the oats are thoroughly cooked and the spices are well combined.
4. Remove from the heat and add the chia seeds and honey/maple syrup (if using).
5. Divide the oats into dishes and garnish with fresh fruit, if preferred.
6. Serve warm and enjoy.

Nutrition Information (per serving):

Calories: 220 Protein: 6g Carbohydrates: 36g Fiber: 7g Sugars: 7g Fat: 6g

Buckwheat Pancakes with Fresh Berries

Prep Time: 10 minutes

Cook Time: 15 minutes

Serve: 2 servings

Ingredients:

- 1/2 cup of buckwheat flour
- 1/4 cup of almond flour
- 1/2 tsp baking powder
- 1/4 tsp baking soda
- 1/2 tsp cinnamon
- 1 tbsp chia seeds (optional)
- 1 cup of unsweetened almond milk
- 1 tsp vanilla extract
- 1 tbsp maple syrup or honey (optional)
- 1 tbsp coconut oil (for cooking)
- 1/2 cup of fresh mixed berries

Instructions:

1. In a medium mixing bowl, combine the buckwheat flour, almond flour, baking powder, baking soda, cinnamon, and chia seeds (if using).
2. Mix the almond milk, vanilla extract, and maple syrup or honey in a separate dish. Slowly pour the wet ingredients into the dry mixture, stirring until mixed.
3. Heat a nonstick pan or griddle over medium heat, then coat with a small quantity of coconut oil.
4. Pour 1/4 cup of batter into the skillet for each pancake. Cook for 2-3 minutes, until bubbles appear on the top, then turn and cook for 1-2 minutes or until golden brown.
5. Repeat with the remaining batter, using extra coconut oil in the skillet as required.
6. Top the pancakes with fresh berries and an optional drizzle of maple syrup.

Nutrition Information (per serving):

Calories: 290 Protein: 8g Carbohydrates: 38g Fiber: 7g Sugars: 8g Fat: 12g

Poached Eggs on a Bed of Sautéed Greens

Prep Time: 5 minutes

Cook Time: 10 minutes

Serve: 2 servings

Ingredients:

- 4 large eggs
- 2 cups of fresh spinach
- 1 tbsp olive oil
- 1 clove garlic, minced
- 1/4 tsp red pepper flakes (optional)
- 1 tbsp lemon juice
- Salt and pepper, to taste
- 2 slices whole grain bread, toasted

Instructions:

1. Fill a medium saucepan with water and heat to a low simmer. Add a touch of vinegar (optional, but it helps with poaching). Crack each egg into a small dish and carefully place one at a time into the boiling water. Cook for approximately 3-4 minutes until the whites are set, but the yolks remain runny. Remove the eggs with a slotted spoon and put aside.
2. While the eggs are poaching, warm the olive oil in a large pan over medium heat. Sauté the minced garlic and red pepper flakes (if using) for approximately a minute or until fragrant.
3. Add the fresh spinach or other leafy greens to the pan and cook for 2-3 minutes or until wilted. Season with lemon juice, salt, and pepper.
4. Divide the sautéed greens into two plates. Place two poached eggs onto each bed of greens.
5. Serve with whole-grain bread on the side for a nutrient-dense breakfast.

Nutrition Information (per serving):

Calories: 220 Protein: 14g Carbohydrates: 7g Fiber: 3g Sugars: 1g Fat: 16g

Banana and Almond Smoothie Bowl

Prep Time: 5 minutes

Cook Time: None

Serve: 1 serving

Ingredients:

- 1 ripe banana, frozen
- 1/4 cup of almond butter (unsweetened)
- 1/2 cup of unsweetened almond milk
- 1 tbsp chia seeds
- 1 tbsp ground flaxseeds
- 1/4 tsp vanilla extract
- A handful of fresh berries (optional for topping)
- 1 tbsp sliced almonds (for topping)
- 1 tbsp unsweetened shredded coconut (for topping)

Instructions:

1. Blend the frozen banana, almond butter, almond milk, chia seeds, flaxseeds, and vanilla extract. Blend until smooth and creamy.
2. Transfer the smoothie mixture to a bowl.
3. Top with fresh berries, sliced almonds, and shredded coconut to add texture and taste.
4. Serve immediately.

Nutrition Information (per serving):

Calories: 350 Protein: 9g Carbohydrates: 40g Fiber: 10g Sugars: 18g Fat: 18g

Millet Porridge with Dried Fruit and Pumpkin Seeds

Prep Time: 5 minutes

Cook Time: 20 minutes

Serve: 2 servings

Ingredients:

- 1/2 cup of millet
- 1 1/2 cups of water or unsweetened almond milk
- 1/4 tsp cinnamon
- 1/4 tsp vanilla extract
- 1 tbsp honey or maple syrup (optional)
- 1/4 cup of dried fruit
- 2 tbsp pumpkin seeds
- A pinch of sea salt
- Fresh fruit (optional for topping)

Instructions:

1. Rinse the millet with cool water. Mix the millet, water (or almond milk), and a sprinkle of sea salt in a medium saucepan. Bring to a boil over medium heat.
2. Reduce the heat to low, cover, and cook for 15-20 minutes until the millet is soft and the liquid has been absorbed.
3. Add the cinnamon, vanilla essence, and honey/maple syrup (if using). Add the dried fruit and let the porridge sit for a minute to absorb the flavors.
4. Divide the porridge into dishes and garnish with pumpkin seeds and fresh fruit, if preferred.
5. Serve warm and enjoy.

Nutrition Information (per serving):

Calories: 280 Protein: 7g Carbohydrates: 44g Fiber: 6g Sugars: 12g Fat: 8g

Sweet Potato Breakfast Bowl with Spinach and Tahini

Prep Time: 10 minutes

Cook Time: 20 minutes

Serve: 2 servings

Ingredients:

- 2 medium sweet potatoes, peeled and cubed
- 1 tbsp olive oil
- 2 cups of fresh spinach, chopped
- 1 clove garlic, minced
- 1 tbsp tahini
- 1 tbsp lemon juice
- 1 tsp maple syrup or honey (optional)
- Salt and pepper, to taste
- 1 tbsp sesame seeds (optional for topping)

Instructions:

1. Preheat the oven to 400 °F (200 °C). Toss the sweet potato cubes with olive oil, salt, and pepper, then lay them equally on a baking sheet. Roast for 20 minutes or until soft and faintly brown, turning halfway through.
2. While the sweet potatoes are roasting, heat a little olive oil in a pan over medium heat. Add the garlic and simmer for approximately 1 minute or until fragrant. Sauté the spinach until wilted, about 2-3 minutes. Season with salt and pepper to taste.
3. In a small mixing bowl, combine the tahini, lemon juice, maple syrup (if using), and a little water to make a smooth, pourable sauce.
4. When the sweet potatoes are done, split them into two dishes. Top with sautéed spinach and sprinkle with tahini.
5. If preferred, sprinkle with sesame seeds. Serve warm.

Nutrition Information (per serving):

Calories: 310 Protein: 5g Carbohydrates: 45g Fiber: 8g Sugars: 10g Fat: 14g

LUNCH RECIPES

Grilled Salmon Salad with Avocado and Lemon Dressing

Prep Time: 10 minutes **Cook Time:** 10 minutes **Serve:** 2 servings

Ingredients:

- 2 salmon fillets
- 1 tbsp olive oil (for grilling)
- Salt and pepper, to taste
- 4 cups of mixed salad greens
- 1 ripe avocado, sliced
- 1/2 cucumber, sliced
- 1/4 cup of cherry tomatoes, halved
- 1 tbsp pumpkin seeds (optional for topping)
- 2 tbsp olive oil
- 1 tbsp lemon juice
- 1 tsp Dijon mustard
- 1 tsp honey or maple syrup (optional)
- Salt and pepper, to taste

Instructions:

1. Preheat the grill or grill pan to medium-high heat. Brush the salmon fillets with olive oil and sprinkle with salt and pepper.
2. Grill the salmon for 4-5 minutes on each side or until it flakes easily with a fork and is well cooked. Set aside to cool somewhat.
3. While the salmon is cooking, make the salad by placing the mixed greens, avocado slices, cucumber, and cherry tomatoes on two plates.
4. Make the dressing in a small bowl by whisking together olive oil, lemon juice, Dijon mustard, honey (if using), salt, and pepper.
5. Once the salmon is cooked, lay one fillet on each salad. Drizzle with lemon dressing and, if preferred, add pumpkin seeds for crunch.
6. Serve immediately and enjoy.

Nutrition Information (per serving):

Calories: 450 Protein: 26g Carbohydrates: 12g Fiber: 7g Sugars: 4g Fat: 34g

Quinoa and Roasted Vegetable Bowl

Prep Time: 10 minutes **Cook Time:** 25 minutes **Serve:** 2 servings

Ingredients:

- 1/2 cup of quinoa, rinsed
- 1 cup of water or vegetable broth
- 1 small zucchini, diced
- 1 red bell pepper, diced
- 1 small sweet potato, peeled and cubed
- 1/2 red onion, diced
- 1 tbsp olive oil
- 1/2 tsp smoked paprika
- 1/2 tsp cumin
- Salt and pepper, to taste
- 1/4 cup of hummus (optional for topping)
- Fresh parsley or cilantro, chopped (optional, for garnish)

Instructions:

1. Preheat the oven to 400 °F (200 °C). Combine the chopped zucchini, red bell pepper, sweet potato, red onion with olive oil, smoked paprika, cumin, salt, and pepper. Spread the veggies on a baking sheet and roast for 20-25 minutes or until soft and faintly caramelized, stirring halfway through.
2. While the veggies roast, prepare the quinoa. Heat 1 cup of water or vegetable broth in a medium saucepan until boiling. Add the rinsed quinoa, decrease the heat to low, cover, and simmer for 15 minutes or until the quinoa is cooked and the liquid has been absorbed. Fluff the quinoa with a fork.
3. Once the veggies are finished, divide the cooked quinoa into two dishes. Top with the roasted veggies.
4. Optional: top with a dollop of hummus and garnish with fresh parsley or cilantro.
5. Serve warm and enjoy.

Nutrition Information (per serving):

Calories: 350 Protein: 9g Carbohydrates: 50g Fiber: 9g Sugars: 10g Fat: 12g

Lentil and Spinach Soup

Prep Time: 10 minutes

Cook Time: 30 minutes

Serve: 4 servings

Ingredients:

- 1 cup of dried lentils, rinsed
- 1 tbsp olive oil
- 1 small onion, diced
- 2 cloves garlic, minced
- 1 carrot, diced
- 1 celery stalk, diced
- 1 tsp ground cumin
- 1/2 tsp turmeric
- 1/4 tsp smoked paprika
- 6 cups of vegetable broth
- 2 cups of fresh spinach, chopped
- 1 tbsp lemon juice
- Salt and pepper, to taste
- Fresh parsley or cilantro, chopped (optional, for garnish)

Instructions:

1. In a large saucepan, warm the olive oil over medium heat. Sauté the chopped onion, garlic, carrot, and celery until softened, about 5-7 minutes.
2. Add the cumin, turmeric, and smoked paprika and simmer for another minute until aromatic.
3. Put the washed lentils and vegetable broth into the pot. Bring the mixture to a boil, lower to a low heat, cover, and cook for 20 minutes, or until the lentils are cooked.
4. Stir in the chopped spinach and simmer for 2-3 minutes or until wilted.
5. Remove the saucepan from the heat and mix in the lemon juice. Season with salt and pepper to taste.
6. Ladle the soup into bowls and top with fresh parsley or cilantro, if preferred.
7. Serve hot, and enjoy this rich, nutritious soup.

Nutrition Information (per serving):

Calories: 220 Protein: 12g Carbohydrates: 35g Fiber: 13g Sugars: 5g Fat: 5g

Turkey and Veggie Lettuce Wraps

Prep Time: 10 minutes

Cook Time: 15 minutes

Serve: 2 servings

Ingredients:

- 8 large lettuce leaves
- 1/2 lb ground turkey (lean)
- 1 tbsp olive oil
- 1 small onion, diced
- 1 clove garlic, minced
- 1/2 red bell pepper, diced
- 1/2 zucchini, diced
- 1 small carrot, shredded
- 2 tbsp soy sauce or tamari (low-sodium)
- 1 tsp fresh ginger, grated
- 1/4 tsp ground black pepper
- 1 tbsp sesame seeds (optional, for garnish)
- Fresh cilantro or parsley, chopped (optional, for garnish)

Instructions:

1. Heat the olive oil in a large pan over medium heat. Sauté the chopped onion and garlic for 2-3 minutes, until aromatic and tender.
2. Add the ground turkey to the skillet and heat, breaking it up with a spoon, until browned and thoroughly cooked, about 5-7 minutes.
3. Combine the chopped red bell pepper, zucchini, and shredded carrot. Cook for a further 3-4 minutes until the veggies are soft.
4. Stir in the soy sauce, grated ginger, and black pepper until well combined. Cook for another 1-2 minutes to let the flavors mix.
5. Remove the skillet from the heat and allow the mixture to cool slightly.
6. To make the wraps, pour the turkey and vegetable mixture onto the center of each lettuce leaf.
7. If preferred, garnish with sesame seeds and chopped fresh cilantro or parsley. Serve immediately and enjoy this light, protein-rich dinner.

Nutrition Information (per serving):

Calories: 280 Protein: 24g Carbohydrates: 10g Fiber: 3g Sugars: 4g Fat: 16g

Chickpea and Cucumber Salad with Tahini Dressing

Prep Time: 10 minutes

Cook Time: None

Serve: 2 servings

Ingredients:

- 1 can (15 oz) chickpeas, drained and rinsed
- 1 cucumber, diced
- 1/2 red onion, finely chopped
- 1/2 cup of cherry tomatoes, halved
- 2 tbsp fresh parsley or cilantro, chopped
- 1 tbsp pumpkin seeds (optional for topping)
- 2 tbsp tahini
- 1 tbsp lemon juice
- 1 tbsp olive oil
- 1 tsp maple syrup or honey (optional)
- 1 clove garlic, minced
- 2-3 tbsp water (to thin the dressing)
- Salt and pepper, to taste

Instructions:

1. Add chickpeas, cucumber, red onion, cherry tomatoes, and chopped parsley or cilantro in a large mixing bowl.
2. In a small mixing bowl, combine tahini, lemon juice, olive oil, maple syrup or honey (if using), chopped garlic, and a touch of salt and pepper. Gradually add water, one tbsp at a time, until the dressing has the appropriate consistency.
3. Pour the tahini dressing over the chickpea-cucumber combination. Toss carefully to coat all of the ingredients equally.
4. If desired, garnish with pumpkin seeds to provide crunch.
5. Serve immediately or chill for up to 2 hours.

Nutrition Information (per serving):

Calories: 320 Protein: 10g Carbohydrates: 36g Fiber: 10g Sugars: 6g Fat: 16g

Baked Cod with Sautéed Greens and Garlic

Prep Time: 10 minutes

Cook Time: 15 minutes

Serve: 2 servings

Ingredients:

- 2 cod fillets (about 4 oz each)
- 1 tbsp olive oil
- 1 tsp lemon zest
- 1 tbsp lemon juice
- 1/2 tsp paprika
- Salt and pepper, to taste
- 2 cups of fresh spinach or kale, chopped
- 2 cloves garlic, minced
- 1 tbsp olive oil (for sautéing)
- 1/4 tsp red pepper flakes (optional)

Instructions:

1. Preheat the oven to 400 °F (200 °C). Line a baking sheet with parchment paper.
2. Mix 1 tbsp olive oil, lemon zest, lemon juice, paprika, salt, and pepper in a small bowl. Apply this mixture equally to the cod fillets.
3. Place the seasoned fish fillets on the prepared baking sheet. Bake in a preheated oven for 12-15 minutes or until the fish is opaque and readily flaked with a fork.
4. While the cod is baking, warm 1 tbsp olive oil in a pan over medium heat. Sauté the minced garlic and red pepper flakes (if using) for approximately a minute or until fragrant.
5. Sauté the spinach or kale in the pan until wilted, about 2-3 minutes. Season with a touch of salt and pepper.
6. When the cod is done, serve it on a dish with the sautéed greens on the side. To add brightness, sprinkle the dish with a little additional lemon juice.

Nutrition Information (per serving):

Calories: 260 Protein: 28g Carbohydrates: 5g Fiber: 2g Sugars: 1g Fat: 14g

Veggie-Loaded Quinoa Stuffed Peppers

Prep Time: 15 minutes **Cook Time:** 30 minutes **Serve:** 4 servings

Ingredients

- 4 large bell peppers (any color), tops cut off and seeds removed
- 1 cup of quinoa, rinsed
- 2 cups of vegetable broth or water
- 1 small onion, diced
- 1 zucchini, diced
- 1 carrot, shredded
- 1/2 cup of cherry tomatoes, halved
- 1/2 cup of corn kernels (fresh or frozen)
- 1 clove garlic, minced
- 1 tbsp olive oil
- 1 tsp cumin
- 1/2 tsp smoked paprika
- Salt and pepper, to taste
- 1/4 cup of fresh parsley or cilantro, chopped (optional, for garnish)

Instructions:

1. Preheat the oven to 375°F (190° C). Lightly butter a baking dish and leave aside.
2. Heat the vegetable broth or water to a boil in a medium saucepan. Add the rinsed quinoa, lower heat to low, cover, and cook for about 15 minutes, or until soft and liquid has been absorbed. Fluff with a fork, then set aside.
3. In a large skillet, heat the olive oil over medium heat. Sauté the onion and garlic for 2-3 minutes, until softened. Cook for 5 minutes, stirring in the zucchini, shredded carrot, cherry tomatoes, and corn until soft.
4. Combine the cooked quinoa, cumin, smoked paprika, salt, and pepper. Mix thoroughly to include all of the flavors.
5. Spoon the quinoa and vegetable mixture into the prepared bell peppers, packing them tightly. Place the filled peppers upright in a prepared baking tray.
6. Cover the baking dish with foil and bake for 25-30 minutes until the peppers are cooked.
7. Remove from the oven and serve with fresh parsley or cilantro, if preferred. Serve warm.

Nutrition Information (per serving):

Calories: 240 Protein: 8g Carbohydrates: 38g Fiber: 8g Sugars: 7g Fat: 7g

Zucchini Noodles with Pesto and Grilled Chicken

Prep Time: 15 minutes

Cook Time: 15 minutes

Serve: 2 servings

Ingredients:

- 2 medium zucchinis, spiralized into noodles
- 2 chicken breasts
- 2 tbsp olive oil (divided)
- Salt and pepper, to taste
- 1/4 cup of homemade or store-bought pesto
- 1 tbsp lemon juice
- 1 tbsp pine nuts (optional for topping)
- Fresh basil leaves (optional, for garnish)

Instructions:

1. Preheat the grill or grill pan to medium-high heat. Add 1 tbsp olive oil to each chicken breast and season with salt and pepper. Grill 5-7 minutes on each side or until the chicken is completely cooked and has reached an internal temperature of 165°F (75°C). Set aside for a few minutes before slicing into strips.
2. While the chicken is cooking, warm the remaining 1 tbsp olive oil in a large pan over medium heat. Add the zucchini noodles and cook for 2-3 minutes or until they soften slightly. Remove from heat.
3. In a large mixing bowl, gently toss the zucchini noodles with the pesto and lemon juice until equally covered.
4. Separate the pesto-coated zucchini noodles between two dishes. Top each platter with grilled chicken pieces.
5. Sprinkle with pine nuts and fresh basil leaves, if preferred. Serve immediately.

Nutrition Information (per serving):

Calories: 360 Protein: 32g Carbohydrates: 8g Fiber: 3g Sugars: 5g Fat: 22g

Curried Cauliflower and Chickpea Stew

Prep Time: 15 minutes

Cook Time: 40 minutes

Serve: 4 servings

Ingredients:

- 1 tbsp olive oil
- 1 large onion, chopped
- 3 cloves garlic, minced
- 1 tbsp grated fresh ginger
- 1 tbsp curry powder
- 1 tsp ground turmeric
- 1 head cauliflower, cut into florets
- 1 can (15 ounces) chickpeas, drained and rinsed
- 1 can (14 ounces) diced tomatoes
- 1 can (14 ounces) coconut milk
- Salt and pepper, to taste
- Fresh cilantro, chopped (for garnish)

Instructions:

1. In a large saucepan, warm the olive oil over medium heat. Sauté the onion until transparent, about 5 minutes.
2. Combine the garlic, ginger, curry powder, and turmeric. Cook for a further minute until fragrant.
3. Place the cauliflower florets, chickpeas, chopped tomatoes, and coconut milk in the saucepan. Stir to mix.
4. Bring the mixture to a boil, then reduce to a simmer, uncovered, for approximately 30 minutes or until the cauliflower is soft.
5. Season with salt and pepper to taste.
6. Garnish with fresh cilantro before serving.

Nutrition Information (per serving):

Calories: 350 Protein: 12g Fat: 20g Carbohydrates: 35g Fiber: 9g Sugar: 8g

Wild Rice and Black Bean Salad with Citrus Dressing

Prep Time: 20 minutes

Cook Time: 45 minutes

Serve: 4 servings

Ingredients:

- 1 cup of wild rice
- 3 cups of water
- 1 can (15 ounces) black beans, rinsed and drained
- 1 red bell pepper, diced
- 1 orange, segmented and chopped
- 1 small red onion, finely chopped
- 1/4 cup of fresh cilantro, chopped
- For the Citrus Dressing:
- 1/4 cup of olive oil
- Juice of 1 lime
- Juice of 1 orange
- 1 tbsp honey (or maple syrup for a vegan option)
- 1 tsp Dijon mustard
- Salt and pepper, to taste

Instructions:

1. Rinse the wild rice in cold water until it is clear. Pour the rice into a medium pot with 3 cups of water. Bring to a boil, then decrease the heat to low, cover, and cook for 45 minutes, or until the rice is cooked and has absorbed the water. Allow it to cool.
2. Add cooled wild rice, black beans, red bell pepper, orange segments, red onion, and cilantro in a large mixing bowl.
3. Combine the olive oil, lime juice, orange juice, honey, and Dijon mustard in a small mixing bowl. Whisk until smooth. Season with salt and pepper to taste.
4. Pour the dressing over the salad and toss to mix.
5. Refrigerate the salad for at least 30 minutes before serving to enable the flavors to combine.

Nutrition Information (per serving):

Calories: 380 Protein: 10g Fat: 15g Carbohydrates: 55g Fiber: 8g Sugar: 10g

Grilled Chicken and Mango Salad with Cilantro Lime Dressing

Prep Time: 20 minutes **Cook Time:** 10 minutes **Serve:** 4 servings

Ingredients

- 4 boneless, skinless chicken breasts
- 1 tbsp olive oil
- Salt and pepper, to taste
- 2 ripe mangoes, peeled and sliced
- 1 avocado, peeled and sliced
- 1/2 red bell pepper, thinly sliced
- 1/4 red onion, thinly sliced
- 1/4 cup of fresh cilantro leaves
- Mixed salad greens (like arugula and romaine)
- For the Cilantro Lime Dressing:
- 1/4 cup of fresh lime juice
- 1/4 cup of olive oil
- 2 tbsp honey
- 2 tbsp chopped fresh cilantro
- 1 garlic clove, minced
- Salt and pepper, to taste

Instructions:

1. Preheat the grill to medium-high heat. Rub olive oil on the chicken breasts and season with salt and pepper. Grill the chicken for 5 minutes per side or until thoroughly cooked, and the internal temperature reaches 165°F (74°C). Let it rest for a few minutes before slicing thinly.
2. In a large salad bowl, combine the mixed greens and top with sliced mango, avocado, red bell pepper, red onion, and grilled chicken.
3. Combine lime juice, olive oil, honey, chopped cilantro, and minced garlic in a small mixing bowl. Season with salt and pepper to taste.
4. Drizzle the dressing over the salad and gently toss to mix.
5. Garnish with fresh cilantro leaves before serving.

Nutrition Information (per serving):

Calories: 450 Protein: 30g Fat: 20g Carbohydrates: 35g Fiber: 5g Sugar: 20g

Roasted Beet and Feta Salad with Walnuts

Prep Time: 15 minutes

Cook Time: 45 minutes

Serve: 4 servings

Ingredients:

- 4 medium beets, peeled and cut into wedges
- 2 tbsp olive oil
- Salt and pepper, to taste
- 1/2 cup of walnut halves
- 1/2 cup of feta cheese, crumbled
- Mixed salad greens (such as arugula and spinach)
- Optional: fresh herbs (like parsley or dill) for garnish
- For the Dressing:
- 3 tbsp balsamic vinegar
- 1 tbsp honey
- 1/3 cup of olive oil
- 1 tsp Dijon mustard
- Salt and pepper, to taste

Instructions:

1. Preheat the oven to 400° F (200° C). Mix the beet wedges with 2 tbsp olive oil, salt, and pepper. Spread on a baking sheet and roast for 45 minutes or until soft and faintly caramelized. Allow them to cool somewhat.
2. Meanwhile, toast the walnut halves in a dry pan over medium heat for 5 minutes, tossing periodically or until lightly browned and aromatic. Set aside for cooling.
3. Add roasted beets, toasted walnuts, crumbled feta, and mixed greens in a large mixing bowl.
4. Combine the balsamic vinegar, honey, olive oil, and Dijon mustard in a small bowl to make the dressing. Season with salt and pepper to taste.
5. Drizzle the dressing over the salad and gently toss to distribute evenly. Garnish with fresh herbs if desired, and serve.

Nutrition Information (per serving):

Calories: 380 Protein: 7g Fat: 30g Carbohydrates: 21g Fiber: 4g Sugar: 15g

Brown Rice Sushi Rolls with Avocado and Cucumber

Prep Time: 30 minutes **Cook Time:** 45 minutes (for the rice) **Serve:** 4 servings

Ingredients:

- 1 cup of brown rice, sushi grade, if available
- 2 cups of water
- 2 tbsp rice vinegar
- 1 tbsp sugar
- 1/2 tsp salt
- 4 sheets nori (dried seaweed)
- 1 cucumber, peeled and cut into long strips
- 1 ripe avocado, peeled, pitted, and sliced
- Optional: soy sauce, wasabi, and pickled ginger for serving

Instructions:

1. Rinse the brown rice in cold water until it is clear. Cook the rinsed rice and water in a rice cooker according to the manufacturer's directions. If cooking on the stove, boil, lower to low heat, cover, and simmer for 45 minutes or until the water has been absorbed and the rice is soft.
2. Mix the rice vinegar, sugar, and salt in a small bowl until dissolved. Gently combine the ingredients into the cooked rice. Spread the rice on a platter or baking sheet to cool until room temperature.
3. Put a sheet of nori on a bamboo sushi mat. Spread 1/4 of the rice evenly over the nori, leaving about 1 inch at the top of the sheet.
4. Place a few strips of cucumber and avocado slices around the rice-covered nori's bottom border.
5. Roll the nori carefully onto the bamboo mat, pressing gently to keep everything in place. To seal the nori edge, use a small amount of water.
6. Cut the roll into six equal pieces using a sharp, moist knife. Repeat with the remaining ingredients, yielding four rolls in total.
7. Optional toppings include soy sauce, wasabi, and pickled ginger.

Nutrition Information (per serving):

Calories: 280 Protein: 4g Fat: 9g Carbohydrates: 46g Fiber: 5g Sugar: 3g

Mediterranean Chickpea and Farro Salad

Prep Time: 15 minutes **Cook Time:** 30 minutes **Serve:** 4 servings

Ingredients:

- 1 cup of farro, rinsed
- 3 cups of water
- 1 can (15 ounces) chickpeas, rinsed and drained
- 1 cup of cherry tomatoes, halved
- 1 cucumber, diced
- 1/2 red onion, thinly sliced
- 1/2 cup of Kalamata olives, pitted and halved
- 1/2 cup of feta cheese, crumbled
- 1/4 cup of fresh parsley, chopped
- For the Dressing:
- 1/4 cup of olive oil
- Juice of 1 lemon
- 2 tbsp red wine vinegar
- 1 tsp dried oregano
- 1 clove garlic, minced
- Salt and pepper, to taste

Instructions:

1. In a medium saucepan, mix the farro and water. Bring to a boil, then decrease the heat to low, cover, and cook for 30 minutes, until farro is cooked and water has been absorbed. Drain the excess water and let the farro to cool.
2. Mix the cooled farro, chickpeas, cherry tomatoes, cucumber, red onion, olives, feta cheese, and parsley in a large salad bowl.
3. In a small mixing bowl, combine olive oil, lemon juice, red wine vinegar, oregano, and minced garlic to make the dressing. Season with salt and pepper to taste.
4. Pour the dressing over the salad and mix thoroughly.
5. Refrigerate the salad before serving to enhance the taste.

Nutrition Information (per serving):

Calories: 400 Protein: 12g Fat: 18g Carbohydrates: 50g Fiber: 10g Sugar: 5g

Spinach and Quinoa Wrap with Hummus

Prep Time: 20 minutes

Cook Time: 15 minutes (for the quinoa)

Serve: 4 servings

Ingredients:

- 1 cup of quinoa
- 2 cups of water
- 4 whole grain or gluten-free wraps
- 1 cup of hummus
- 2 cups of fresh spinach leaves
- 1 red bell pepper, thinly sliced
- 1 carrot, grated
- 1/2 cucumber, thinly sliced
- 1/4 cup of red onion, thinly sliced
- Salt and pepper, to taste

Instructions:

1. Rinse the quinoa in cool running water until it is clear. In a medium saucepan, combine the quinoa and water. Bring to a boil. Reduce the heat to low, cover, and cook for 15 minutes or until the water is absorbed. Remove from fire and let stand for 5 minutes before fluffing with a fork and allow to cool.
2. Arrange the wraps on a clean surface. Fill each wrap with a thick amount of hummus.
3. Layer the cooked quinoa, fresh spinach leaves, sliced bell pepper, grated carrot, sliced cucumber, and red onion across the wraps.
4. Season with salt and pepper to taste.
5. Carefully roll up the wraps, tucking the edges in as you go to produce a tight roll.
6. Cut each wrap in half diagonally and serve immediately, or wrap in foil to preserve fresh for later.

Nutrition Information (per serving):

Calories: 370 Protein: 12g Fat: 14g Carbohydrates: 53g Fiber: 9g Sugar: 4g

DINNER RECIPES

Baked Salmon with Roasted Brussels sprouts

Prep Time: 10 minutes

Cook Time: 25 minutes

Serve: 4 servings

Ingredients:

- 4 salmon fillets (about 4-6 ounces each)
- 1 tbsp olive oil
- 1 tbsp lemon juice
- 2 cloves garlic, minced
- 1 tsp dried oregano
- Salt and pepper, to taste
- 1 pound Brussels sprouts, trimmed and halved
- 2 tbsp olive oil (for Brussels sprouts)
- 1 tsp balsamic vinegar
- Optional: lemon wedges for serving

Instructions:

1. Preheat the oven to 400 °F (200 °C). Line a baking sheet with parchment or foil.
2. Place the salmon fillets on one side of the baking sheet. Drizzle with 1 tbsp olive oil and lemon juice. Season with minced garlic, oregano, salt, and pepper. Set aside.
3. Mix the halved Brussels sprouts in a separate bowl with 2 tbsp olive oil, balsamic vinegar, salt, and pepper.
4. Spread the Brussels sprouts on the other side of the baking sheet in a single layer.
5. Bake the salmon and Brussels sprouts for 20-25 minutes, or until the fish is fully cooked and easily flaked with a fork and the Brussels sprouts are golden and crispy.
6. Serve the salmon beside the roasted Brussels sprouts, garnished with lemon wedges if preferred.

Nutrition Information (per serving):

Calories: 420 Protein: 35g Fat: 24g Carbohydrates: 15g Fiber: 6g Sugar: 3g

Grilled Chicken Breast with Sweet Potato Mash

Prep Time: 15 minutes **Cook Time:** 30 minutes **Serve:** 4 servings

Ingredients:

- For the Grilled Chicken:
- 4 boneless, skinless chicken breasts
- 2 tbsp olive oil
- 1 tbsp lemon juice
- 2 garlic cloves, minced
- 1 tsp dried thyme
- 1 tsp dried rosemary
- Salt and pepper, to taste
- For the Sweet Potato Mash:
- 3 large sweet potatoes, peeled and cubed
- 2 tbsp olive oil or butter (for a richer mash)
- 1/4 cup of unsweetened almond milk (or regular milk)
- Salt and pepper, to taste
- Optional: a pinch of cinnamon or nutmeg

Instructions:

1. Whisk the olive oil, lemon juice, garlic, thyme, rosemary, salt, and pepper in a small bowl.
2. Allow the chicken breasts to marinate for at least 10 minutes.
3. Preheat the grill or grill pan to medium-high heat. Grill the chicken breasts on each side for 6-7 minutes until thoroughly cooked and the internal temperature reaches 165°F (74°C).
4. Allow the chicken to rest for a few minutes before serving.
5. While the chicken is cooking, cook the sweet potato cubes in a large saucepan of salted water. Bring to a boil, then simmer for 15-20 minutes or until the potatoes are soft when pricked with a fork.
6. Drain the potatoes, then return them to the saucepan. Combine olive oil (or butter) with almond milk. Mash until smooth and creamy. Season with salt, pepper, and a touch of cinnamon or nutmeg, if preferred.
7. Plate the grilled chicken with the sweet potato mash and enjoy!

Nutrition Information (per serving):

Calories: 420 Protein: 35g Fat: 15g Carbohydrates: 40g Fiber: 7g

Turmeric-Ginger Chicken Stir-Fry with Vegetables

Prep Time: 15 minutes

Cook Time: 20 minutes

Serve: 4

Ingredients:

- 1 lb (450g) boneless, skinless chicken breast, thinly sliced
- 1 tbsp olive oil
- 1 tsp ground turmeric
- 1 tbsp fresh ginger, grated
- 2 garlic cloves, minced
- 1 medium red bell pepper, sliced
- 1 medium yellow bell pepper, sliced
- 1 cup of broccoli florets
- 1 medium carrot, thinly sliced
- 1 tbsp low-sodium soy sauce or coconut aminos
- 1 tbsp lemon juice
- 1/4 tsp black pepper
- 1/4 tsp salt (optional)
- 2 green onions, chopped (for garnish)

Instructions:

1. Mix the chicken pieces, turmeric, ginger, and garlic in a large bowl. Mix well to coat the chicken evenly.
2. Heat the olive oil in a large pan or wok over medium-high heat. Cook the chicken for 5-7 minutes or until browned and cooked.
3. Place the sliced bell peppers, broccoli florets, and carrot in the skillet. Stir fry for 5-7 minutes or until the veggies are soft and crisp.
4. Add the soy sauce (or coconut aminos), lemon juice, black pepper, and salt (if desired). Cook for 2-3 minutes, stirring regularly, until well mixed.
5. Before serving, remove from heat and garnish with finely chopped green onions.

Nutrition Information (per serving):

Calories: 210 Protein: 28g Fat: 7g Carbohydrates: 9g Fiber: 3g Sugar: 4g Sodium: 320mg

Lentil and Vegetable Shepherd's Pie

Prep Time: 20 minutes **Cook Time:** 45 minutes **Serve:** 4

Ingredients

- 1 cup of dried green or brown lentils
- 1 tbsp olive oil
- 1 medium onion, diced
- 2 garlic cloves, minced
- 1 medium carrot, diced
- 1 celery stalk, diced
- 1 cup of mushrooms, sliced
- 1 cup of vegetable broth, low-sodium
- 1 tbsp tomato paste
- 1 tsp dried thyme
- 1 tsp dried rosemary
- 1 cup of frozen peas
- 4 medium potatoes, peeled and cubed (for the topping)
- ¼ cup of unsweetened almond milk (or other plant-based milk)
- 1 tbsp olive oil (for the mashed potatoes)
- Salt and pepper to taste

Instructions

1. Rinse the lentils and put them in a saucepan with three cups of water. Bring to a boil, then decrease the heat and simmer for 20-25 minutes or until the lentils are cooked. Drain and set aside.
2. While the lentils simmer, heat 1 tbsp olive oil in a large skillet over medium heat. Sauté the chopped onion and garlic for 2-3 minutes, until softened.
3. Cook for 5 minutes or until the carrots, celery, and mushrooms soften.
4. Combine the tomato paste, thyme, rosemary, and vegetable broth. Bring the mixture to a simmer and cook for approximately 10 minutes to enable the flavors to combine.
5. Once the veggies are soft, mix in the cooked lentils and frozen peas. Stir in the salt and pepper to taste. Allow the mixture to boil for another 5 minutes.
6. While the filling simmers, cook the potatoes in a large saucepan of water until tender (10-12 minutes). Drain potatoes and mash with ¼ cup of almond milk and 1 tbsp olive oil. Season with salt and pepper to taste.
7. Preheat the oven to 375° Fahrenheit (190° Celsius). Spread the lentil and veggie mixture equally on a baking dish. Cover with mashed potatoes, spreading them evenly over the contents.

8. Place the baking dish in an oven for 20 minutes or until the top is golden brown and the filling bubbles.
9. Allow the Shepherd's Pie to cool for a few minutes before serving.

Nutrition Information (per serving):

Calories: 320 Protein: 13g Carbohydrates: 55g Dietary Fiber: 12g Sugars: 5g Fat: 8g

Quinoa-Stuffed Bell Peppers with Black Beans

Prep Time: 15 minutes **Cook Time:** 35 minutes **Serve:** 4

Ingredients:

- 4 large bell peppers (any color), tops cut off and seeds removed
- 1 cup of cooked quinoa
- 1 tbsp olive oil
- 1 small onion, diced
- 2 garlic cloves, minced
- 1 cup of black beans, cooked
- 1 cup of diced tomatoes
- 1 tsp ground cumin
- 1 tsp smoked paprika
- 1 tsp dried oregano
- Salt and pepper to taste
- ½ cup of fresh cilantro, chopped (optional)
- ½ cup of shredded dairy-free cheese

Instructions:

1. Preheat the oven to 375° Fahrenheit (190° Celsius). Lightly butter a baking dish and leave aside.
2. In a large skillet, heat the olive oil over medium heat. Sauté the chopped onion and garlic for 2-3 minutes, until tender and aromatic.
3. Add the cooked quinoa, black beans, diced tomatoes, cumin, smoked paprika, oregano, salt, and pepper to the pan. Stir well to mix, then heat for 5 minutes to let the flavors mingle.
4. Remove from the fire and add the fresh cilantro (if using).
5. Stuff each bell pepper with the quinoa and black bean mixture, pushing it down to fill fully.

6. Place the filled peppers upright in the prepared baking dish. If desired, sprinkle the tops with shredded dairy-free cheese.
7. Cover with foil and bake in the oven for 25-30 minutes or until the peppers are cooked.
8. Remove the foil and bake for 5 minutes until the tops are gently browned.
9. Allow the stuffed peppers to cool slightly before serving.

Nutrition Information (per serving):

Calories: 270 Protein: 10g Carbohydrates: 45g Dietary Fiber: 12g Sugars: 6g Fat: 7g

Baked Cod with Lemon and Garlic Green Beans

Prep Time: 10 minutes **Cook Time:** 20 minutes **Serve:** 4

Ingredients:

- 4 cod fillets (about 4-6 oz each)
- 2 tbsp olive oil
- 3 garlic cloves, minced
- 1 lemon, sliced
- 1 tbsp lemon juice
- 1 tsp dried thyme
- Salt and pepper to taste
- 1 lb green beans, trimmed
- 1 tbsp olive oil (for green beans)
- ½ tsp garlic powder
- ½ tsp lemon zest

Instructions:

1. Preheat the oven to 400 °F (200 °C). Cover a baking sheet with parchment paper or gently oil it.
2. Place the fish fillets on one side of the baking sheet. Drizzle 2 tbsp olive oil over the fillets and season with garlic, dry thyme, salt, and pepper. Garnish each fillet with lemon slices and drizzle with lemon juice.
3. On the other side of the baking sheet, place the green beans. Drizzle 1 tbsp olive oil over the green beans, then season with garlic powder, lemon zest, salt, and pepper. Toss to coat evenly.
4. Place the baking sheet in the oven for 15-20 minutes until the fish is flaky and opaque and the green beans are cooked through.

5. Once finished, remove the baking sheet from the oven. Serve the fish fillets with the roasted green beans as a side.

Nutrition Information (per serving):

Calories: 290 Protein: 30g Carbohydrates: 12g Dietary Fiber: 4g Sugars: 3g Fat: 12g

Grilled Tofu and Veggie Skewers with Brown Rice

Prep Time: 15 minutes **Cook Time:** 30 minutes **Serve:** 4

Ingredients:

- 1 block of firm tofu, drained and cubed
- 2 tbsp olive oil
- 1 tbsp soy sauce (low sodium)
- 1 tbsp lemon juice
- 1 tsp garlic powder
- 1 tsp smoked paprika
- 1 red bell pepper, cut into chunks
- 1 yellow bell pepper, cut into chunks
- 1 zucchini, sliced
- 1 red onion, cut into wedges
- 1 cup of cherry tomatoes
- 1 cup of brown rice
- Salt and pepper to taste
- Fresh parsley, chopped (optional, for garnish)

Instructions:

1. Cook the brown rice according to the package instructions. Once finished, set aside.
2. Combine the olive oil, soy sauce, lemon juice, garlic powder, and smoked paprika in a bowl. Add salt and pepper to taste. Toss the tofu cubes in the marinade to coat evenly, then set aside for 10 minutes.
3. Preheat the grill or grill pan to medium heat.
4. Thread the marinated tofu, bell peppers, zucchini, onion, and cherry tomatoes onto skewers.
5. Grill the skewers for 10-12 minutes, flipping them regularly, until the veggies are cooked and the tofu is gently browned.

6. Serve the grilled tofu and vegetable skewers on a bed of brown rice. Garnish with fresh parsley if preferred.

Nutrition Information (per serving):

Calories: 320 Protein: 12g Carbohydrates: 45g Dietary Fiber: 6g Sugars: 6g Fat: 12g

Chickpea and Spinach Curry with Cauliflower Rice

Prep Time: 15 minutes **Cook Time:** 25 minutes **Serve:** 4

Ingredients

- 1 tbsp olive oil
- 1 small onion, diced
- 2 garlic cloves, minced
- 1-inch piece of fresh ginger, grated
- 1 tbsp curry powder
- 1 tsp ground cumin
- 1 tsp turmeric
- 1 can (15 oz) chickpeas, drained and rinsed
- 1 can (14 oz) diced tomatoes, no salt added
- 1 cup of coconut milk, light
- 4 cups of fresh spinach, chopped
- Salt and pepper to taste
- 1 head cauliflower, grated into rice-sized pieces
- 1 tbsp olive oil (for cauliflower rice)
- Fresh cilantro, chopped (optional, for garnish)

Instructions:

1. In a large skillet, heat 1 tbsp olive oil over medium heat. Sauté the diced onion for 3-4 minutes, until softened.
2. Cook for another minute, stirring in the minced garlic and grated ginger until fragrant.
3. Cook for 1 minute to toast the curry powder, cumin, and turmeric.
4. Place the chickpeas, chopped tomatoes, and coconut milk in the pan. Stir well to mix. Bring to a simmer and cook for 10-12 minutes, allowing the flavors to combine.
5. Stir in the fresh spinach and simmer for 2-3 minutes or until wilted. Season with salt and pepper to taste.

6. While the curry simmer, warm 1 tbsp olive oil in a separate skillet over medium heat. Sauté the grated cauliflower for 5-7 minutes, until soft. Season with salt and pepper to taste.
7. Serve the chickpea and spinach stew on a bed of cauliflower rice. Garnish with fresh cilantro if desired.

Nutrition Information (per serving):

Calories: 280 Protein: 9g Carbohydrates: 30g Dietary Fiber: 9g Sugars: 8g Fat: 14g

Turkey Meatballs with Zucchini Noodles and Tomato Sauce

Prep Time: 15 minutes **Cook Time:** 30 minutes **Serve:** 4

Ingredients:

- For the Turkey Meatballs:
- 1 lb ground turkey
- 1 egg, beaten
- ½ cup of almond flour
- 2 garlic cloves, minced
- 1 tsp dried oregano
- 1 tsp dried basil
- Salt and pepper to taste
- 2 tbsp olive oil (for frying)
- For the Tomato Sauce:
- 1 tbsp olive oil
- 1 small onion, diced
- 2 garlic cloves, minced
- 1 can (14 oz) crushed tomatoes, no salt added
- 1 tsp dried basil
- 1 tsp dried oregano
- Salt and pepper to taste
- For the Zucchini Noodles:
- 4 medium zucchinis, spiralized into noodles
- 1 tbsp olive oil
- Salt and pepper to taste

Instructions:

1. Add ground turkey, beaten egg, almond flour, chopped garlic, oregano, basil, salt, and pepper in a large mixing bowl. Mix until well mixed. Roll the mixture into tiny meatballs.
2. Heat 2 tbsp olive oil in a large pan over medium heat. Cook the turkey meatballs for 8-10 minutes, flipping regularly, until they are browned on both sides and cooked. Remove from the skillet and put aside.
3. Heat 1 tbsp olive oil in the same skillet and sauté the chopped onion for 2-3 minutes, until softened. Add the minced garlic and simmer for another minute until fragrant.
4. Combine the smashed tomatoes, basil, oregano, salt, and pepper. Allow the sauce to boil to blend the flavors for 10-12 minutes. Adjust the seasoning as required.
5. While the sauce is simmering, heat 1 tbsp olive oil in a separate skillet over medium heat. Sauté the zucchini noodles for 3-5 minutes, until soft but firm. Season with salt and pepper to taste.
6. Serve the turkey meatballs over a bed of zucchini noodles, topped with tomato sauce.

Nutrition Information (per serving):

Calories: 340 Protein: 27g Carbohydrates: 18g Dietary Fiber: 5g Sugars: 8g Fat: 18g

Lemon-garlic shrimp with Roasted Asparagus

Prep Time: 10 minutes

Cook Time: 20 minutes

Serve: 4

Ingredients

- For the Shrimp:
- 1 lb shrimp, peeled and deveined
- 2 tbsp olive oil
- 3 garlic cloves, minced
- 1 lemon, juiced and zested
- 1 tsp dried parsley (or fresh, chopped)
- Salt and pepper to taste
- For the Roasted Asparagus:
- 1 lb asparagus, trimmed
- 1 tbsp olive oil

- Salt and pepper to taste
- 1 tsp garlic powder

Instructions:

1. Preheat the oven to 400 °F (200 °C). Place the trimmed asparagus on a baking sheet and sprinkle with 1 tbsp olive oil. Season with garlic powder, salt, and pepper. Toss to coat evenly.
2. Roast the asparagus in a warm oven for 12-15 minutes until tender and slightly crisp at the tips. Remove from the oven and put aside.
3. While the asparagus roasts, warm 2 tbsp olive oil in a large pan over medium heat. Sauté the minced garlic for 1 minute, until fragrant.
4. Add the shrimp to the skillet and cook for 2-3 minutes per side or until pink and cooked through.
5. Add the lemon juice and zest to the pan when the shrimp are done. Add the dried parsley and season with salt and pepper to taste. Cook for one further minute, letting the flavors combine.
6. Serve the roasted asparagus beside the lemon-garlic shrimp, garnished with more lemon slices if preferred.

Nutrition Information (per serving):

Calories: 220 Protein: 25g Carbohydrates: 7g Dietary Fiber: 3g Sugars: 2g Fat: 10g

Moroccan-spiced vegetable Tagine with Couscous

Prep Time: 15 minutes

Cook Time: 35 minutes

Serve: 4

Ingredients:

- 1 tbsp olive oil
- 1 onion, diced
- 3 garlic cloves, minced
- 1-inch piece fresh ginger, grated
- 2 carrots, peeled and sliced
- 1 zucchini, chopped
- 1 red bell pepper, chopped
- 1 cup of butternut squash, cubed
- 1 can (15 oz) chickpeas, drained and rinsed
- 1 can (14 oz) diced tomatoes, no salt added
- 1 cup of vegetable broth, low-sodium
- 1 tsp ground cumin
- 1 tsp ground cinnamon
- 1 tsp ground turmeric
- ½ tsp ground paprika
- ½ tsp ground coriander
- Salt and pepper to taste
- ¼ cup of raisins (optional)
- Fresh cilantro, chopped (for garnish)
- For the Couscous:
- 1 cup of couscous
- 1 cup of vegetable broth or water
- 1 tbsp olive oil
- Salt to taste

Instructions:

1. Heat the olive oil over medium heat in a large saucepan or tagine. Sauté the diced onion, garlic, and grated ginger for 3-4 minutes, until softened.

2. Put the carrots, zucchini, red bell pepper, and butternut squash into the saucepan. To toast them, cook for 2 minutes, stirring in the cumin, cinnamon, turmeric, paprika, and coriander.
3. Pour in the chopped tomatoes, veggie broth, and chickpeas. Stir until fully combined, then bring to a simmer. Cover and simmer for 25–30 minutes, stirring periodically, until the veggies are cooked.
4. In the last 5 minutes of cooking, add the raisins (if using) and season with salt and pepper.
5. While the tagine is cooking, bring 1 cup of vegetable broth or water to a boil in a small saucepan. Remove from the fire and mix in the couscous, 1 tbsp olive oil, and a sprinkle of salt. Cover and let aside for 5 minutes, then fluff with a fork.
6. Serve the Moroccan-spiced vegetable tagine with couscous. Garnish with fresh cilantro.

Nutrition Information (per serving):

Calories: 360 Protein: 10g Carbohydrates: 65g Dietary Fiber: 12g Sugars: 14g Fat: 10g

Herb-Roasted Chicken with Root Vegetables

Prep Time: 15 minutes **Cook Time:** 1 hour **Serve:** 4

Ingredients:

- For the Chicken:
- 4 bone-in, skin-on chicken thighs (or breasts)
- 2 tbsp olive oil
- 2 tsp dried thyme
- 2 tsp dried rosemary
- 2 garlic cloves, minced
- 1 lemon, juiced and zested
- Salt and pepper to taste
- For the Root Vegetables:
- 2 large carrots, peeled and chopped
- 2 parsnips, peeled and chopped
- 1 large sweet potato, peeled and cubed
- 1 red onion, cut into wedges
- 2 tbsp olive oil
- 1 tsp dried thyme
- 1 tsp dried rosemary
- Salt and pepper to taste

Instructions:

1. Preheat the oven to 400 °F (200 °C). Line a large baking sheet with parchment paper or gently oil it.
2. In a small mixing bowl, combine olive oil, minced garlic, lemon juice, lemon zest, dried thyme, and rosemary. Season the chicken thighs with salt and pepper, then apply the herb mixture evenly to the chicken.
3. In a large mixing bowl, combine the carrots, parsnips, sweet potato, red onion with the olive oil, dried thyme, dry rosemary, salt, and pepper.
4. Place the seasoned chicken thighs and root vegetables in a single layer on the prepared baking sheet. Place the baking sheet in the oven and roast for 45-50 minutes until the chicken is thoroughly cooked (internal temperature of 165°F) and the veggies are soft and caramelized.
5. After the chicken and veggies have been cooked, remove them from the oven and let them rest for a few minutes. Serve the herb-roasted chicken with roasted root vegetables.

Nutrition Information (per serving):

Calories: 420 Protein: 25g Carbohydrates: 30g Dietary Fiber: 7g Sugars: 8g Fat: 23g

Grilled Eggplant with Chickpea Salad

Prep Time: 15 minutes

Cook Time: 10 minutes

Serve: 4

Ingredients:

- For the Grilled Eggplant:
- 2 large eggplants, sliced into ½-inch rounds
- 2 tbsp olive oil
- 1 tsp ground cumin
- 1 tsp smoked paprika
- Salt and pepper to taste
- For the Chickpea Salad:
- 1 can (15 oz) chickpeas, drained and rinsed
- 1 cup of cherry tomatoes, halved
- 1 small cucumber, diced

- 1 small red onion, finely diced
- ¼ cup of fresh parsley, chopped
- 2 tbsp olive oil
- 1 tbsp lemon juice
- 1 tsp ground cumin
- Salt and pepper to taste

Instructions:

1. Preheat the grill or grill pan to medium heat. Combine olive oil, ground cumin, smoked paprika, salt, and pepper in a small bowl. Brush both sides of the eggplant slices with seasoned olive oil.
2. Grill the eggplant slices for 4-5 minutes per side or until soft and with excellent grill marks. Remove off the grill and put aside.
3. Add chickpeas, cherry tomatoes, cucumber, red onion, and fresh parsley in a large mixing bowl.
4. Combine the olive oil, lemon juice, ground cumin, salt, and pepper in a small mixing bowl. Toss the chickpea salad with the dressing until combined.
5. Place the grilled eggplant slices on a serving plate, then top with the chickpea salad. Garnish with more parsley if desired.

Nutrition Information (per serving):

Calories: 290 Protein: 6g Carbohydrates: 28g Dietary Fiber: 10g Sugars: 6g

Seared Tuna with a Quinoa and Kale Salad

Prep Time: 15 minutes **Cook Time:** 10 minutes **Serve:** 4

Ingredients:

- For the Seared Tuna:
- 4 tuna steaks (about 6 oz each)
- 2 tbsp olive oil
- 1 tbsp soy sauce (low sodium)
- 1 tbsp lemon juice
- 1 tsp sesame seeds
- Salt and pepper to taste
- For the Quinoa and Kale Salad:
- 1 cup of quinoa, rinsed
- 2 cups of water or vegetable broth (low sodium)
- 4 cups of fresh kale, chopped
- 1 cup of cherry tomatoes, halved
- 1 small cucumber, diced
- ¼ cup of red onion, finely diced
- 2 tbsp olive oil
- 1 tbsp lemon juice
- 1 tsp Dijon mustard
- Salt and pepper to taste

Instructions:

1. Heat 2 cups of water or vegetable broth in a medium saucepan until boiling. Add the quinoa, decrease the heat, and cook for 15 minutes or until the liquid has been absorbed. Fluff with a fork, then set aside.
2. Combine 2 tbsp olive oil, soy sauce, lemon juice, and sesame seeds in a small bowl. Season the tuna steaks with salt and pepper, then brush both sides with the marinade.
3. Preheat a large skillet or grill pan to medium-high heat. Add the tuna steaks and sear for 2 minutes on each side for medium-rare, or longer if preferred. Remove from the heat and put aside.
4. Add cooked quinoa, chopped kale, cherry tomatoes, cucumber, and red onion in a large mixing bowl.
5. In a small bowl, combine 2 tbsp olive oil, 1 tbsp lemon juice, Dijon mustard, salt, and pepper. Toss the quinoa and kale salad with the dressing until combined.
6. Serve the seared tuna steaks with the quinoa and kale salad. Drizzle with the leftover dressing if desired.

Nutrition Information (per serving):

Calories: 400 Protein: 35g Carbohydrates: 30g Dietary Fiber: 6g Sugars: 5g Fat: 16g Fat: 18g

Spaghetti Squash with Pesto and Roasted Vegetables

Prep Time: 15 minutes **Cook Time:** 45 minutes **Serve:** 4

Ingredients:

- 1 large spaghetti squash, halved and seeds removed
- 1 tbsp olive oil
- Salt and pepper to taste
- For the Pesto:
- 2 cups of fresh basil leaves
- ¼ cup of pine nuts (or walnuts)
- 2 garlic cloves
- ¼ cup of olive oil
- 2 tbsp lemon juice
- ¼ cup of nutritional yeast or Parmesan cheese
- Salt and pepper to taste
- 1 zucchini, chopped
- 1 red bell pepper, chopped
- 1 yellow bell pepper, chopped
- 1 red onion, sliced
- 1 tbsp olive oil
- 1 tsp dried oregano
- Salt and pepper to taste

Instructions:

1. Preheat the oven to 400 °F (200 °C). Drizzle olive oil on the cut sides of the spaghetti squash and season with salt and pepper. Place the squash halves cut side down on a baking sheet. Roast in a preheated oven for 35-40 minutes or until the flesh is soft and readily scraped with a fork.
2. While the squash roasts, combine the diced zucchini, bell peppers, and red onion with olive oil, oregano, salt, and pepper. Place the veggies on a separate baking sheet and roast for 20-25 minutes or until soft and faintly caramelized.

3. Blend the fresh basil, pine nuts, garlic, olive oil, lemon juice, and nutritional yeast (or Parmesan cheese) in a food processor. Blend until smooth, adding a bit extra olive oil if required. Season with salt and pepper to taste.
4. Once the spaghetti squash has been cooked, use a fork to scrape the flesh into spaghetti-like strands. Toss the squash strands in the pesto until well coated.
5. Divide the pesto-coated spaghetti squash across dishes and top with the roasted veggies. If desired, garnish with more basil or nutritional yeast.

Nutrition Information (per serving):

Calories: 300 Protein: 6g Carbohydrates: 28g Dietary Fiber: 8g Sugars: 9g Fat: 20g

Baked Tilapia with Sautéed Spinach and Mushrooms

Prep Time: 10 minutes **Cook Time:** 20 minutes **Serve:** 4

Ingredients:

- 4 tilapia fillets
- 2 tbsp olive oil
- 1 tbsp lemon juice
- 1 tsp garlic powder
- 1 tsp dried thyme
- Salt and pepper to taste
- 1 tbsp olive oil
- 1 small onion, diced
- 2 garlic cloves, minced
- 2 cups of mushrooms, sliced
- 4 cups of fresh spinach
- Salt and pepper to taste
- 1 tbsp lemon juice

Instructions:

1. Preheat the oven to 400 °F (200 °C). Cover a baking sheet with parchment paper or gently oil it.
2. Place the tilapia fillets on the prepared baking sheet. Drizzle with olive oil and lemon juice, then season with garlic powder, thyme, salt, and pepper. Bake for 12-15 minutes or until the fish is readily flaked with a fork.

3. While the tilapia is baking, warm 1 tbsp olive oil in a large pan over medium heat. Sauté the diced onion for 2-3 minutes, until softened.
4. Cook the minced garlic and sliced mushrooms in the pan for another 5 minutes or until the mushrooms are soft.
5. Add the fresh spinach and simmer for 2-3 minutes or until wilted. Season with salt, pepper, and 1 tbsp lemon juice. Stir well and remove from heat.
6. Serve the baked tilapia with sautéed spinach and mushrooms.

Nutrition Information (per serving):

Calories: 280 Protein: 30g Carbohydrates: 8g Dietary Fiber: 3g Sugars: 3g Fat: 14g

Black Bean and Sweet Potato Enchiladas

Prep Time: 20 minutes **Cook Time:** 30 minutes **Serve:** 4

Ingredients:

- For the Filling:
- 2 medium sweet potatoes, peeled and diced
- 1 tbsp olive oil
- 1 small onion, diced
- 2 garlic cloves, minced
- 1 can (15 oz) black beans, drained and rinsed
- 1 tsp ground cumin
- 1 tsp chili powder
- ½ tsp smoked paprika
- Salt and pepper to taste
- ½ cup of fresh cilantro, chopped (optional)
- For the Enchiladas:
- 8 small corn tortillas
- 1 can (15 oz) enchilada sauce
- 1 cup of dairy-free shredded cheese (optional)
- 1 tbsp olive oil (for greasing the baking dish)

Instructions:

1. Preheat the oven to 375° Fahrenheit (190° Celsius). Lightly coat a baking dish with olive oil and leave aside.

2. In a large skillet, heat 1 tbsp olive oil over medium heat. Sauté the diced sweet potatoes for 8-10 minutes or until tender. Remove the sweet potatoes from the pan and put them aside.
3. In the same pan, sauté the diced onion and garlic for 2-3 minutes or until softened. Combine the black beans, cooked sweet potatoes, cumin, chili powder, smoked paprika, salt, and pepper. Stir well and heat for a further 5 minutes to enable the flavors to combine. Remove from the heat and whisk in the chopped cilantro if using.
4. Warm the maize tortillas slightly to make them more flexible. Spoon the sweet potato and black bean mixture onto each tortilla, wrap it up, and lay it seam side down in the buttered baking dish.
5. Pour the enchilada sauce evenly over the filled tortillas, then top with dairy-free shredded cheese if preferred.
6. Bake the enchiladas in a preheated oven for 20-25 minutes or until the sauce bubbles and the cheese (if used) melts.
7. Serve hot, topped with more cilantro or avocado slices if preferred.

Nutrition Information (per serving):

Calories: 380 Protein: 12g Carbohydrates: 65g Dietary Fiber: 14g Sugars: 10g Fat: 9g

Black Bean and Sweet Potato Enchiladas

Prep Time: 20 minutes **Cook Time:** 30 minutes **Serve:** 4

Ingredients:

- For the Filling:
- 2 medium sweet potatoes, peeled and diced
- 1 tbsp olive oil
- 1 small onion, diced
- 2 garlic cloves, minced
- 1 can (15 oz) black beans, drained and rinsed
- 1 tsp ground cumin
- 1 tsp chili powder
- ½ tsp smoked paprika
- Salt and pepper to taste
- ½ cup of fresh cilantro, chopped (optional)
- For the Enchiladas:
- 8 small corn tortillas
- 1 can (15 oz) enchilada sauce

- 1 cup of dairy-free shredded cheese (optional)
- 1 tbsp olive oil (for greasing the baking dish)

Instructions:

1. Preheat the oven to 375° Fahrenheit (190° Celsius). Lightly coat a baking dish with olive oil and leave aside.
2. In a large skillet, heat 1 tbsp olive oil over medium heat. Sauté the diced sweet potatoes for 8-10 minutes or until tender. Remove the sweet potatoes from the pan and put them aside.
3. In the same pan, sauté the diced onion and garlic for 2-3 minutes or until softened. Combine the black beans, cooked sweet potatoes, cumin, chili powder, smoked paprika, salt, and pepper. Stir well and heat for a further 5 minutes to enable the flavors to combine. Remove from the heat and whisk in the chopped cilantro if using.
4. Warm the maize tortillas slightly to make them more flexible. Spoon the sweet potato and black bean mixture onto each tortilla, wrap it up, and lay it seam side down in the buttered baking dish.
5. Pour the enchilada sauce evenly over the filled tortillas, then top with dairy-free shredded cheese if preferred.
6. Bake the enchiladas in a preheated oven for 20-25 minutes or until the sauce bubbles and the cheese (if used) melts.
7. Serve hot, topped with more cilantro or avocado slices if preferred.

Nutrition Information (per serving):

Calories: 380 Protein: 12g Carbohydrates: 65g Dietary Fiber: 14g Sugars: 10g Fat: 9g

Roasted Turkey Breast with Mashed Cauliflower

Prep Time: 15 minutes **Cook Time:** 1 hour **Serve:** 4

Ingredients:

- 1 small boneless turkey breast
- 2 tbsp olive oil
- 2 garlic cloves, minced
- 1 tsp dried thyme
- 1 tsp dried rosemary
- 1 tsp paprika
- Salt and pepper to taste
- 1 lemon, sliced
- 1 large head of cauliflower, cut into florets
- 2 tbsp olive oil
- 2 garlic cloves, minced
- ¼ cup of unsweetened almond milk
- Salt and pepper to taste
- Fresh parsley, chopped

Instructions:

1. Preheat the oven to 375° Fahrenheit (190° Celsius). Put the turkey breast in a roasting pan. In a small bowl, combine olive oil, minced garlic, thyme, rosemary, paprika, salt, and pepper. Rub the mixture all over the turkey breast. Place the lemon slices on top of the turkey.
2. Cook the turkey breast in a preheated oven for 45-60 minutes or until the internal temperature reaches 165°F (74°C). Allow the turkey to rest for ten minutes before slicing.
3. While the turkey roasts, heat a large pot of water to a boil. Cook the cauliflower florets for 10-12 minutes or until soft. Drain and set aside.
4. In a large skillet, heat 2 tbsp olive oil over medium heat. Sauté the minced garlic for 1-2 minutes, until aromatic.
5. Add the cooked cauliflower to the pan and mash with a potato masher or immersion blender for a smoother texture. Add the almond milk and season with salt and pepper to suit.
6. Topped with fresh parsley, serve the roasted turkey breast with the mashed cauliflower.

Nutrition Information (per serving):

Calories: 320 Protein: 30g Carbohydrates: 12g Dietary Fiber: 5g Sugars: 3g Fat: 18g

Tempeh Stir-Fry with Broccoli and Peppers

Prep Time: 15 minutes **Cook Time:** 15 minutes **Serve:** 4

Ingredients:

- 1 block (8 oz) tempeh, cut into bite-sized cubes
- 2 tbsp olive oil, divided
- 2 tbsp soy sauce (low sodium)
- 1 tbsp rice vinegar
- 1 tbsp maple syrup or honey
- 2 garlic cloves, minced
- 1 tsp fresh ginger, grated
- 1 large red bell pepper, sliced
- 1 large yellow bell pepper, sliced
- 2 cups of broccoli florets
- ¼ cup of water (for steaming)
- 1 tbsp sesame oil (optional for flavor)
- Sesame seeds, for garnish
- Fresh cilantro or green onions, chopped (optional, for garnish)

Instructions:

1. Combine 1 tbsp of olive oil, soy sauce, rice vinegar, maple syrup, garlic, and ginger in a small mixing bowl. Add the cubed tempeh and toss to coat. Allow it to marinade for ten minutes while you prepare the veggies.
2. Heat 1 tbsp olive oil in a large pan or wok over medium heat. Cook the marinated tempeh for 5-6 minutes, stirring regularly, until golden brown on both sides. Remove from the pan and put aside.
3. In the same pan, combine the broccoli florets and sliced bell pepper. Stir-fry for 3–4 minutes. Cover the pan, add ¼ cup of water, and steam the veggies for 2-3 minutes until soft yet crisp.
4. Return the tempeh to the skillet with the veggies. Drizzle with sesame oil (if using) and mix everything. Cook for another 2 minutes to blend the flavors.
5. Serve the tempeh stir-fry with sesame seeds and, if preferred, fresh cilantro or green onions as garnish.

Nutrition Information (per serving):

Calories: 270 Protein: 14g Carbohydrates: 20g Dietary Fiber: 6g Sugars: 7g Fat: 15g

SMOOTHIES AND DRINKS

Blueberry-Spinach Smoothie with Chia Seeds

Prep Time: 5 minutes

Cook Time: N/A

Serving: 1

Ingredients

- 1 cup of fresh spinach leaves
- ½ cup of frozen blueberries
- 1 tbsp chia seeds
- ½ cup of unsweetened almond milk
- 1 tbsp almond butter
- 1 tsp honey
- ¼ tsp ground cinnamon
- 4-5 ice cubes

Instructions:

1. Blend the spinach, blueberries, chia seeds, almond milk, almond butter, honey (if using), and cinnamon.
2. Add the ice cubes and process on high until smooth and creamy.
3. Pour into a glass and drink immediately.

Nutrition Information (per serving):

Calories: 220 Protein: 6g Carbohydrates: 25g Fat: 12g Fiber: 8g Sugar: 10g

Almond Butter Banana Smoothie

Prep Time: 5 minutes

Cook Time: N/A

Serving: 1

Ingredients:

- 1 ripe banana
- 1 tbsp almond butter
- 1 tbsp ground flaxseeds
- ½ cup of unsweetened almond milk
- ½ tsp vanilla extract
- ¼ tsp ground cinnamon
- 4-5 ice cubes

Instructions:

1. Add the banana, almond butter, ground flaxseeds, almond milk, vanilla extract, and cinnamon to a blender.
2. Combine the ice cubes and mix until smooth and creamy.
3. Pour into a glass and drink immediately.

Nutrition Information (per serving):

Calories: 250 Protein: 6g Carbohydrates: 32g Fat: 12g Fiber: 6g Sugar: 14g

Pineapple and Kale Anti-Inflammatory Smoothie

Prep Time: 5 minutes

Cook Time: N/A

Serving: 1

Ingredients

- 1 cup of fresh kale leaves (stems removed)
- ½ cup of frozen pineapple chunks
- ½ cup of unsweetened coconut water
- 1 tbsp fresh lemon juice
- 1 tsp grated fresh ginger
- 1 tbsp chia seeds
- ½ tsp turmeric powder
- 4-5 ice cubes

Instructions:

1. Blend the kale, pineapple, coconut water, lemon juice, ginger, chia seeds, and turmeric powder.
2. Add the ice cubes and process until smooth and thoroughly blended.
3. Pour into a glass and serve immediately.

Nutrition Information (per serving):

Calories: 150 Protein: 3g Carbohydrates: 30g Fat: 4g Fiber: 7g Sugar: 16g

Turmeric Latte with Almond Milk

Prep Time: 5 minutes

Cook Time: 5 minutes

Serving: 1

Ingredients:

- 1 cup of unsweetened almond milk
- ½ tsp ground turmeric
- ¼ tsp ground cinnamon
- ¼ tsp ground ginger
- 1 tsp honey or maple syrup
- Pinch of black pepper
- ½ tsp vanilla extract
- 1 tbsp coconut oil

Instructions:

1. Heat the almond milk over medium heat in a small saucepan until it is warm but not boiling.
2. Combine the turmeric, cinnamon, ginger, black pepper, vanilla essence, and honey or maple syrup (if desired).
3. Stir for about 3-5 minutes or until the mixture is thoroughly blended and heated.
4. If using coconut oil, combine it with the ingredients and whisk until frothy.
5. Pour the turmeric latte into a cup and serve warm.

Nutrition Information (per serving):

Calories: 100 Protein: 2g Carbohydrates: 10g Fat: 6g Fiber: 1g Sugar: 5g

Strawberry and Avocado Smoothie

Prep Time: 5 minutes

Cook Time: N/A

Serving: 1

Ingredients:

- ½ ripe avocado
- 1 cup of frozen strawberries
- ½ cup of unsweetened almond milk
- 1 tbsp chia seeds
- 1 tsp honey or maple syrup
- ½ tsp vanilla extract
- 4-5 ice cubes

Instructions:

1. Blend the avocado, frozen strawberries, almond milk, chia seeds, honey (if using), and vanilla essence.
2. Combine the ice cubes and mix until smooth and creamy.
3. Pour into a glass and drink immediately.

Nutrition Information (per serving):

Calories: 230 Protein: 4g Carbohydrates: 26g Fat: 14g Fiber: 9g Sugar: 12g

Green Tea and Ginger Elixir

Prep Time: 5 minutes

Cook Time: 5 minutes

Serving: 1

Ingredients:

- 1 cup of hot water
- 1 green tea bag
- 1 tsp freshly grated ginger
- 1 tsp honey or maple syrup (optional)
- 1 tbsp fresh lemon juice
- ¼ tsp ground turmeric
- Pinch of black pepper

Instructions:

1. Boil the water and pour it into a cup. Add the green tea bag and brew for 3-4 minutes.
2. Remove the tea bag, then add the freshly grated ginger, honey (if using), lemon juice, turmeric, and black pepper.
3. Stir well to integrate all ingredients, and let the ginger and turmeric infuse the tea.
4. Drink warm for a calming and anti-inflammatory boost.

Nutrition Information (per serving):

Calories: 20 Protein: 0g Carbohydrates: 5g Fat: 0g Fiber: 0g Sugar: 4g

Mixed Berry and Flaxseed Smoothie

Prep Time: 5 minutes

Cook Time: N/A

Serving: 1

Ingredients:

- 1 cup of mixed frozen berries
- 1 tbsp ground flaxseeds
- ½ cup of unsweetened almond milk (or any plant-based milk)
- ½ cup of plain Greek yogurt
- 1 tsp honey or maple syrup
- ½ tsp vanilla extract
- 4-5 ice cubes

Instructions:

1. Add mixed berries, ground flaxseeds, almond milk, Greek yogurt, honey (if desired), and vanilla extract in a blender.
2. Combine the ice cubes and mix until smooth and creamy.
3. Pour into a glass and drink immediately.

Nutrition Information (per serving):

Calories: 190 Protein: 6g Carbohydrates: 26g Fat: 7g Fiber: 8g Sugar: 16g

Carrot and Ginger Juice with Lemon

Prep Time: 10 minutes

Cook Time: N/A

Serving: 1

Ingredients

- 3 medium carrots, peeled and chopped
- 1-inch piece of fresh ginger, peeled
- 1 tbsp fresh lemon juice
- ½ cup of water
- 1 tsp honey or maple syrup
- Ice cubes (optional)

Instructions

1. Add the carrots, ginger, and water to a blender.
2. Blend until smooth, adding extra water to get the desired consistency.
3. Strain the juice into a glass using a fine mesh strainer or cheesecloth, pressing firmly to get all the liquid.
4. Add the fresh lemon juice and honey (if using).
5. Alternatively, serve cooled with ice cubes.

Nutrition Information (per serving):

Calories: 80 Protein: 1g Carbohydrates: 20g Fat: 0g Fiber: 5g Sugar: 10g

Coconut Water with Fresh Berries and Mint

Prep Time: 5 minutes

Cook Time: N/A

Serving: 1

Ingredients

- 1 cup of coconut water
- ½ cup of fresh mixed berries
- 4-5 fresh mint leaves
- 1 tsp fresh lime juice (optional)
- Ice cubes (optional)

Instructions:

1. In a glass, combine the fresh mixed berries and mint leaves.
2. To unleash the flavors, gently mix the berries and mint leaves. Pour coconut water over the mixed mixture.
3. If desired, add fresh lime juice to enhance the flavor.
4. Stir and serve cold, with ice cubes if desired.

Nutrition Information (per serving):

Calories: 60 Protein: 0g Carbohydrates: 15g Fat: 0g Fiber: 3g Sugar: 10g

Orange-Turmeric Smoothie with Chia Seeds

Prep Time: 5 minutes

Cook Time: N/A

Serving: 1

Ingredients:

- 1 large orange, peeled and segmented
- ½ banana, frozen
- ½ tsp ground turmeric
- 1 tbsp chia seeds
- ½ cup of unsweetened almond milk (or any plant-based milk)
- 1 tsp honey or maple syrup (optional for sweetness)
- 4-5 ice cubes

Instructions:

1. Mix orange segments, frozen bananas, turmeric, chia seeds, and almond milk in a blender.
2. Add the honey or maple syrup (if using) and ice cubes.
3. Blend until smooth and creamy.
4. Pour into a glass and serve immediately.

Nutrition Information (per serving):

Calories: 200 Protein: 4g Carbohydrates: 42g Fat: 5g Fiber: 9g Sugar: 27g

SNACKS AND APPETIZERS

Roasted Chickpeas with Paprika

Prep Time: 5 minutes

Cook Time: 30 minutes

Serving: 2

Ingredients:

- 1 can (15 oz) chickpeas, drained and rinsed
- 1 tbsp olive oil
- 1 tsp smoked paprika
- ½ tsp garlic powder
- ½ tsp ground cumin
- ¼ tsp sea salt
- ¼ tsp black pepper

Instructions:

1. Preheat the oven to 400 degrees Fahrenheit (200 degrees Celsius) and line a baking sheet with parchment paper.
2. To remove extra moisture, pat the chickpeas dry with a paper towel.
3. Toss the chickpeas with olive oil, smoked paprika, garlic powder, cumin, salt, and black pepper until equally covered.
4. Place the chickpeas in a single layer on the prepared baking sheet.
5. Roast the chickpeas in a preheated oven for 25-30 minutes, stirring the pan halfway through, until crispy and golden brown.
6. Remove from the oven and allow to cool slightly before serving.

Nutrition Information (per serving):

Calories: 180 Protein: 6g Carbohydrates: 24g Fat: 7g Fiber: 6g Sugar: 1g

Veggie Sticks with Hummus

Prep Time: 10 minutes

Cook Time: N/A

Serving: 2

Ingredients:

- For the Veggie Sticks:
- 1 large carrot, cut into sticks
- 1 cucumber, cut into sticks
- 1 red bell pepper, sliced
- 1 celery stalk, cut into sticks
- For the Hummus:
- 1 can (15 oz) chickpeas, drained and rinsed
- 2 tbsp tahini
- 1 tbsp olive oil
- 1 tbsp fresh lemon juice
- 1 garlic clove, minced
- ¼ tsp ground cumin
- ¼ tsp salt
- 2-3 tbsp water (to reach desired consistency)

Instructions:

1. Blend chickpeas, tahini, olive oil, lemon juice, garlic, cumin, and salt in a food processor.
2. Blend until smooth, then add water one spoonful at a time until you achieve the desired consistency.
3. Taste and adjust the seasoning as required.
4. Place the carrot, cucumber, bell pepper, and celery sticks on a serving platter.
5. Serve the vegetable sticks with hummus for dipping.

Nutrition Information (per serving):

Calories: 220 Protein: 6g Carbohydrates: 26g Fat: 11g Fiber: 8g Sugar: 5g

Avocado-Stuffed Cucumber Boats

Prep Time: 10 minutes

Cook Time: N/A

Serving: 2

Ingredients:

- 1 large cucumber, halved lengthwise and seeds scooped out
- 1 ripe avocado
- 1 tbsp fresh lemon juice
- 1 tbsp chopped fresh cilantro (optional)
- ¼ tsp garlic powder
- Salt and pepper to taste
- Cherry tomatoes, halved (for garnish)

Instructions:

1. In a bowl, mash the avocado with a fork.
2. Stir in the lemon juice, cilantro (if using), garlic powder, salt, and pepper until well blended.
3. Spoon the avocado mixture into the hollowed-out cucumber halves.
4. Garnish with halved cherry tomatoes.
5. Serve immediately.

Nutrition Information (per serving):

Calories: 150 Protein: 2g Carbohydrates: 10g Fat: 13g Fiber: 7g Sugar: 3g

Almond-Coconut Energy Bites

Prep Time: 10 minutes

Cook Time: N/A

Serving: 10 bites

Ingredients:

- 1 cup of rolled oats
- ½ cup of almond butter
- ¼ cup of shredded unsweetened coconut
- 2 tbsp chia seeds
- 2 tbsp ground flaxseeds
- 2 tbsp honey or maple syrup
- 1 tsp vanilla extract
- ¼ tsp ground cinnamon
- 1-2 tbsp water (if needed)

Instructions:

1. Mix the rolled oats, almond butter, shredded coconut, chia seeds, ground flaxseeds, honey, vanilla essence, and cinnamon in a medium bowl.
2. Mix until the ingredients are completely mixed. If the mixture is too dry, add 1 tbsp until it comes together.
3. Scoop off 1 tbsp of the mixture and form it into a ball with your palms.
4. Repeat with the remaining ingredients to make approximately 10 energy bites.
5. Put the energy bites in the refrigerator for 30 minutes to firm up.
6. Enjoy as a fast snack or refrigerate in an airtight container for up to a week.

Nutrition Information (per serving):

Calories: 120 Protein: 4g Carbohydrates: 12g Fat: 7g Fiber: 4g Sugar: 5g

Sweet Potato Chips with Guacamole

Prep Time: 10 minutes

Cook Time: 25 minutes

Serving: 2

Ingredients:

- For the Sweet Potato Chips:
- 1 large sweet potato, thinly sliced
- 1 tbsp olive oil
- ¼ tsp paprika
- ¼ tsp garlic powder
- Salt and pepper to taste
- For the Guacamole:
- 1 ripe avocado
- 1 tbsp fresh lime juice
- 1 small garlic clove, minced
- 1 tbsp chopped fresh cilantro (optional)
- Salt and pepper to taste

Instructions:

1. Preheat the oven to 400 degrees Fahrenheit (200 degrees Celsius) and line a baking sheet with parchment paper.
2. In a mixing bowl, combine the sweet potato slices with the olive oil, paprika, garlic powder, salt, and pepper.
3. Place the slices in a single layer on the baking pan.
4. Bake the chips for 20-25 minutes, turning halfway through, until crispy and golden brown.
5. Remove from the oven and allow to cool slightly before serving. In a mixing bowl, mash the avocado with a fork until smooth.
6. Combine the lime juice, garlic, cilantro (if using), salt, and pepper. Serve the sweet potato chips with guacamole for dipping.

Nutrition Information (per serving):

Calories: 250 Protein: 3g Carbohydrates: 30g Fat: 14g Fiber: 8g Sugar: 5g

Baked Zucchini Fries with Spicy Yogurt Dip

Prep Time: 10 minutes **Cook Time:** 20 minutes Serving: 2

Ingredients:

- For the Zucchini Fries:
- 2 medium zucchinis, cut into fry-like strips
- ½ cup of whole wheat breadcrumbs
- ¼ cup of grated Parmesan cheese (optional)
- 1 tsp garlic powder
- 1 tsp smoked paprika
- 1 large egg, beaten
- Salt and pepper to taste
- For the Spicy Yogurt Dip:
- ½ cup of plain Greek yogurt
- 1 tsp hot sauce (adjust to taste)
- 1 tsp fresh lemon juice
- ½ tsp garlic powder
- Salt and pepper to taste

Instructions:

1. Preheat the oven to 425°F (220°C). Line a baking sheet with parchment paper.
2. In a shallow bowl, combine the breadcrumbs, parmesan cheese (if using), garlic powder, smoked paprika, salt, and pepper.
3. Dip each zucchini strip into the beaten egg, then coat it with the breadcrumb mixture, gently pressing it to adhere.
4. Place the coated zucchini fries in a single layer on the prepared baking sheet.
5. Bake the fries for 15-20 minutes, turning halfway through, until golden brown and crispy.
6. Remove from the oven and allow to cool slightly before serving.
7. Combine Greek yogurt, spicy sauce, lemon juice, garlic powder, salt, and pepper in a small mixing bowl.
8. Serve the cooked zucchini fries with a spicy yogurt dip on the side.

Nutrition Information (per serving):

Calories: 220 Protein: 9g Carbohydrates: 22g Fat: 10g Fiber: 4g Sugar: 4g

Greek Yogurt with Walnuts and Honey

Prep Time: 5 minutes

Cook Time: N/A

Serving: 1

Ingredients:

- 1 cup of plain Greek yogurt (or dairy-free yogurt)
- 2 tbsp chopped walnuts
- 1 tbsp honey
- ¼ tsp ground cinnamon (optional)

Instructions:

1. Spoon the Greek yogurt into a bowl.
2. Garnish with chopped walnuts and sprinkle with honey.
3. For extra taste, sprinkle with ground cinnamon.
4. Serve immediately and enjoy.

Nutrition Information (per serving):

Calories: 250 Protein: 12g Carbohydrates: 20g Fat: 12g Fiber: 2g Sugar: 16g

Kale Chips with Nutritional Yeast

Prep Time: 10 minutes

Cook Time: 15 minutes

Serving: 2

Ingredients:

- 1 bunch of kale, stems removed and leaves torn into bite-sized pieces
- 1 tbsp olive oil
- 2 tbsp nutritional yeast
- ¼ tsp garlic powder
- Salt and pepper to taste

Instructions:

1. Preheat the oven to 350°F/175°C and line a baking sheet with parchment paper.
2. Toss the kale with olive oil in a large mixing bowl, ensuring the leaves are equally covered.
3. Sprinkle the nutritional yeast, garlic powder, salt, and pepper over the kale and toss to combine.
4. Place the kale in a single layer on the prepared baking sheet.
5. Bake for 12–15 minutes or until the kale is crispy but not burnt. Keep an eye on it to avoid overcooking.
6. Remove from the oven and allow to cool slightly before serving.

Nutrition Information (per serving):

Calories: 120 Protein: 4g Carbohydrates: 7g Fat: 8g Fiber: 2g Sugar: 0g

Apple Slices with Almond Butter and Cinnamon

Prep Time: 5 minutes

Cook Time: N/A

Serving: 1

Ingredients:

- 1 medium apple, cored and sliced
- 2 tbsp almond butter
- ¼ tsp ground cinnamon
- 1 tsp chia seeds

Instructions:

1. Place the apple slices on a plate.
2. Drizzle or spread almond butter over the apple slices.
3. Sprinkle with ground cinnamon and chia seeds, if desired.
4. Serve immediately for a fast, nutritious snack.

Nutrition Information (per serving):

Calories: 210 Protein: 4g Carbohydrates: 28g Fat: 11g Fiber: 6g Sugar: 18g

Baked Beet Chips with Tahini Dip

Prep Time: 10 minutes

Cook Time: 25 minutes

Serving: 2

Ingredients:

- For the Beet Chips:
- 2 medium beets, peeled and thinly sliced
- 1 tbsp olive oil
- ¼ tsp sea salt
- ¼ tsp black pepper
- For the Tahini Dip:
- 2 tbsp tahini
- 1 tbsp fresh lemon juice
- 1 tbsp water (to thin the dip)
- 1 small garlic clove, minced
- ¼ tsp ground cumin
- Salt and pepper to taste

Instructions:

1. Preheat the oven to 375°F (190°C), then line a baking sheet with parchment paper.
2. Toss the beet slices in olive oil, salt, and pepper until thoroughly covered.
3. Place the slices in a single layer on the baking pan.
4. Bake for 20-25 minutes, turning halfway through or until the chips are crispy. Keep an eye on things to avoid getting heated.
5. Remove from the oven and allow to cool before serving. Combine the tahini, lemon juice, water, garlic, cumin, salt, and pepper in a small mixing bowl.
6. If necessary, add additional water to get the desired consistency. Serve beet chips with the tahini dip.

Nutrition Information (per serving):

Calories: 180 Protein: 4g Carbohydrates: 17g Fat: 11g Fiber: 5g Sugar: 9g

Edamame with Sea Salt and Lemon

Prep Time: 5 minutes

Cook Time: 5 minutes

Serving: 2

Ingredients:

- 1 cup of frozen edamame (in pods)
- 1 tbsp sea salt
- 1 tbsp fresh lemon juice
- Lemon wedges (for garnish)

Instructions:

1. Bring a saucepan of water to a boil before adding the frozen edamame. Cook for 4–5 minutes or until tender.
2. Drain the edamame and place in a serving dish.
3. Garnish with sea salt and fresh lemon juice. Toss to coat evenly, then garnish with lemon wedges.
4. Serve warm for a light and refreshing snack.

Nutrition Information (per serving):

Calories: 120 Protein: 10g Carbohydrates: 10g Fat: 4g Fiber: 4g Sugar: 2g

Sliced Veggies with Sunflower Seed Pâté

Prep Time: 10 minutes

Cook Time: N/A

Serving: 2

Ingredients:

- For the Sunflower Seed Pâté:
- ½ cup of raw sunflower seeds (soaked in water for 2-3 hours and drained)
- 1 tbsp fresh lemon juice
- 1 tbsp olive oil
- 1 small garlic clove, minced
- 1 tbsp fresh parsley, chopped
- ¼ tsp ground cumin
- Salt and pepper to taste
- 2-3 tbsp water (to reach desired consistency)
- For the Sliced Veggies:
- 1 cucumber, sliced
- 1 red bell pepper, sliced
- 1 carrot, cut into sticks
- 1 celery stalk, cut into sticks

Instructions:

1. Blend the soaked and drained sunflower seeds in a food processor with lemon juice, olive oil, garlic, parsley, cumin, salt, and pepper.
2. Process until smooth, then add water one spoonful at a time until you achieve the desired consistency.
3. Taste and adjust the seasoning as required. Place the cucumber, bell pepper, carrot, and celery sticks on a serving platter.
4. Serve the cut vegetables with sunflower seed pâté for dipping.

Nutrition Information (per serving):

Calories: 180 Protein: 6g Carbohydrates: 12g Fat: 12g Fiber: 5g Sugar: 5g

Baked Carrot Fries with Curry Dip

Prep Time: 10 minutes

Cook Time: 25 minutes

Serving: 2

Ingredients:

- For the Carrot Fries:
- 4 large carrots, peeled and cut into thin strips
- 1 tbsp olive oil
- ½ tsp smoked paprika
- ½ tsp garlic powder
- Salt and pepper to taste
- For the Curry Dip:
- ½ cup of plain Greek yogurt (or dairy-free yogurt)
- 1 tsp curry powder
- 1 tsp fresh lemon juice
- Salt and pepper to taste

Instructions:

1. Preheat the oven to 400 degrees Fahrenheit (200 degrees Celsius) and line a baking sheet with parchment paper.
2. Toss the carrot strips with olive oil, smoked paprika, garlic powder, salt, and pepper until well combined.
3. Place the carrot fries in a single layer on the baking pan.
4. Bake for 20-25 minutes, rotating halfway through or until the fries are soft and slightly crunchy around the edges.
5. Remove from the oven and allow it to cool slightly. Combine Greek yogurt, curry powder, lemon juice, salt, and pepper in a small mixing bowl.
6. Serve the baked carrot fries with a side of curry dip.

Nutrition Information (per serving):

Calories: 160 Protein: 5g Carbohydrates: 20g Fat: 7g Fiber: 6g Sugar: 10g

Cucumber and Radish Salad with Lemon Vinaigrette

Prep Time: 10 minutes

Cook Time: N/A

Serving: 2

Ingredients:

- For the Salad:
- 1 cucumber, thinly sliced
- 5-6 radishes, thinly sliced
- 2 tbsp fresh parsley, chopped
- 1 tbsp fresh dill, chopped (optional)
- For the Lemon Vinaigrette:
- 2 tbsp fresh lemon juice
- 1 tbsp olive oil
- ½ tsp Dijon mustard
- 1 tsp honey or maple syrup (optional)
- Salt and pepper to taste

Instructions:

1. In a large mixing bowl, combine the cucumbers, radishes, parsley, and dill (if using).
2. In a small mixing bowl, combine the lemon juice, olive oil, Dijon mustard, honey (if using), salt, and pepper until thoroughly blended.
3. Toss the cucumber and radish salad with the lemon vinaigrette until evenly coated.
4. Serve immediately as a light, refreshing side dish.

Nutrition Information (per serving):

Calories: 90 Protein: 1g Carbohydrates: 7g Fat: 6g Fiber: 2g Sugar: 3g

Mini Stuffed Bell Peppers with Hummus

Prep Time: 10 minutes

Cook Time: N/A

Serving: 4

Ingredients:

- 10-12 mini bell peppers, halved and seeds removed
- 1 cup of hummus
- 1 tbsp fresh parsley, chopped
- 1 tsp paprika (optional, for garnish)
- 1 tbsp olive oil (optional for drizzling)

Instructions:

1. Wash and split the small bell peppers, then remove the seeds.
2. Place roughly 1 spoonful of hummus in each bell pepper half. Place the stuffed peppers on a serving platter.
3. Garnish with chopped parsley, paprika, and olive oil, if preferred.
4. Serve immediately as a nutritious snack or appetizer.

Nutrition Information (per serving):

Calories: 100 Protein: 4g Carbohydrates: 12g Fat: 5g Fiber: 4g Sugar: 4g

SIDES AND SALADS

Roasted Brussels sprouts with Balsamic Glaze

Prep Time: 10 minutes

Cook Time: 25 minutes

Serving: 4

Ingredients

- 1 lb Brussels sprouts, trimmed and halved
- 2 tbsp olive oil
- Salt and pepper to taste
- ¼ cup of balsamic vinegar
- 1 tbsp honey or maple syrup (optional)

Instructions:

1. Preheat the oven to 400 degrees Fahrenheit (200 degrees Celsius) and line a baking sheet with parchment paper.
2. Combine Brussels sprouts, olive oil, salt, and pepper in a large mixing bowl.
3. Place the Brussels sprouts in a single layer on the prepared baking sheet.
4. Roast for 20-25 minutes, rotating halfway through or until the sprouts are brown and crispy around the edges.
5. While the Brussels sprouts are roasting, make the balsamic glaze. Bring the balsamic vinegar and honey (if using) to a simmer over medium heat in a small saucepan. Cook for 5-7 minutes, stirring regularly, until the liquid has reduced and thickened into a glaze.
6. Remove the Brussels sprouts from the oven and sprinkle them with the balsamic glaze.
7. Serve immediately as a tasty side dish.

Nutrition Information (per serving):

Calories: 130 Protein: 3g Carbohydrates: 12g Fat: 7g Fiber: 4g Sugar: 6g

Quinoa and Cucumber Salad with Lemon Dressing

Prep Time: 10 minutes

Cook Time: 15 minutes (for quinoa)

Serving: 4

Ingredients:

- For the Salad:
- 1 cup of quinoa, rinsed
- 2 cups of water
- 1 large cucumber, diced
- ½ cup of cherry tomatoes, halved
- 2 tbsp fresh parsley, chopped
- 1 tbsp fresh mint, chopped (optional)
- For the Lemon Dressing:
- 3 tbsp fresh lemon juice
- 2 tbsp olive oil
- 1 tsp Dijon mustard
- 1 tsp honey or maple syrup (optional)
- Salt and pepper to taste

Instructions:

1. In a medium saucepan, mix the quinoa and water. Bring to a boil, then decrease the heat to low and cover. Simmer for approximately 15 minutes until the water is absorbed and the quinoa is fluffy.
2. Remove from heat, fluff the quinoa with a fork, and let cool slightly.
3. In a large mixing bowl, add the cooked quinoa, chopped cucumber, cherry tomatoes, parsley, and mint (if desired).
4. In a small mixing bowl, combine the lemon juice, olive oil, Dijon mustard, honey (if using), salt, and pepper until thoroughly blended.
5. Pour the lemon dressing over the quinoa and toss to coat evenly.
6. Serve chilled or at room temperature for a light and refreshing salad.

Nutrition Information (per serving):

Calories: 180 Protein: 5g Carbohydrates: 25g Fat: 7g Fiber: 4g Sugar: 3g

Sautéed Kale with Garlic and Lemon

Prep Time: 5 minutes

Cook Time: 10 minutes

Serving: 2

Ingredients:

- 1 bunch kale, stems removed and leaves roughly chopped
- 1 tbsp olive oil
- 2 garlic cloves, minced
- 1 tbsp fresh lemon juice
- Salt and pepper to taste
- Lemon wedges (for garnish)

Instructions:

1. Heat the olive oil in a large pan over medium heat.
2. Sauté the minced garlic for 1-2 minutes, until aromatic, taking care not to burn it.
3. Toss the chopped kale in the pan with the garlic and oil.
4. Cook for 5-7 minutes, stirring periodically, until the kale has wilted and softened.
5. Remove from heat and add the fresh lemon juice. Season with salt and pepper to taste.
6. Serve immediately, topped with lemon slices for added taste.

Nutrition Information (per serving):

Calories: 100 Protein: 3g Carbohydrates: 8g Fat: 7g Fiber: 3g Sugar: 1g

Grilled Asparagus with Lemon Zest

Prep Time: 5 minutes

Cook Time: 10 minutes

Serving: 2

Ingredients:

- 1 bunch asparagus, trimmed
- 1 tbsp olive oil
- Zest of 1 lemon
- 1 tbsp fresh lemon juice
- Salt and pepper to taste

Instructions:

1. Preheat the grill or grill pan to medium-high heat. Toss the asparagus with olive oil, salt, and pepper until well combined.
2. Grill the asparagus on each side for 3-5 minutes until tender and slightly browned. Remove the asparagus from the grill and place on a serving platter.
3. Drizzle with fresh lemon juice and garnish with lemon zest.
4. Serve immediately as a light and refreshing side dish.

Nutrition Information (per serving):

Calories: 80 Protein: 3g Carbohydrates: 7g Fat: 6g Fiber: 3g Sugar: 2g

Roasted Sweet Potatoes with Cinnamon and Olive Oil

Prep Time: 5 minutes

Cook Time: 25 minutes

Serving: 2

Ingredients:

- 2 medium sweet potatoes, peeled and cubed
- 1 tbsp olive oil
- 1 tsp ground cinnamon
- Salt and pepper to taste

Instructions:

1. Preheat the oven to 400 degrees Fahrenheit (200 degrees Celsius) and line a baking sheet with parchment paper.
2. Combine the sweet potato cubes, olive oil, cinnamon, salt, and pepper in a large mixing bowl.
3. Spread the sweet potatoes in a single layer on the prepared baking sheet.
4. Roast the sweet potatoes in a preheated oven for 20-25 minutes, turning halfway through, until soft and golden brown.
5. Remove from the oven and allow to cool slightly before serving.

Nutrition Information (per serving):

Calories: 180 Protein: 2g Carbohydrates: 33g Fat: 5g Fiber: 5g Sugar: 7g

Wild Rice Pilaf with Cranberries and Almonds

Prep Time: 10 minutes

Cook Time: 45 minutes

Serving: 4

Ingredients:

- 1 cup of wild rice, rinsed
- 2 cups of vegetable broth (or water)
- ½ cup of dried cranberries
- ¼ cup of slivered almonds toasted
- 1 tbsp olive oil
- 1 small onion, finely chopped
- 1 garlic clove, minced
- 1 tbsp fresh parsley, chopped (optional)
- Salt and pepper to taste

Instructions:

1. In a medium saucepan, heat the vegetable broth (or water) to a boil. Add the washed wild rice, decrease the heat to low, cover, and cook for 40-45 minutes or until cooked and the liquid has been absorbed.
2. While the rice is cooking, warm the olive oil in a pan over medium heat. Sauté the chopped onion and garlic until the onion is transparent, about 5 minutes.
3. When the rice is finished, fluff it with a fork before transferring it to a large bowl.
4. Combine the sautéed onions and garlic, dried cranberries, toasted almonds, and fresh parsley (if using).
5. Season with salt and pepper to taste. Serve warm as a tasty side dish or a light supper.

Nutrition Information (per serving):

Calories: 250 Protein: 5g Carbohydrates: 38g Fat: 8g Fiber: 4g Sugar: 7g

Cabbage Slaw with Apple and Carrot

Prep Time: 10 minutes

Cook Time: N/A

Serving: 4

Ingredients:

- 2 cups of green cabbage, finely shredded
- 1 large apple, julienned
- 1 large carrot, grated
- 2 tbsp apple cider vinegar
- 1 tbsp olive oil
- 1 tsp honey or maple syrup
- 1 tbsp fresh lemon juice
- Salt and pepper to taste
- 1 tbsp fresh parsley, chopped (optional)

Instructions:

1. Add the shredded cabbage, julienned apples, and grated carrot in a large mixing bowl.
2. Combine the apple cider vinegar, olive oil, honey or maple syrup, lemon juice, salt, and pepper in a small mixing bowl.
3. Pour the dressing over the cabbage mixture and toss to evenly coat.
4. Garnish with fresh parsley if desired.
5. Serve immediately or chill for up to an hour to enable the flavors to combine.

Nutrition Information (per serving):

Calories: 90 Protein: 1g Carbohydrates: 15g Fat: 4g Fiber: 4g Sugar: 9g

Spinach Salad with Strawberries and Pecans

Prep Time: 10 minutes

Cook Time: N/A

Serving: 2

Ingredients:

- 4 cups of fresh baby spinach
- 1 cup of fresh strawberries, sliced
- ¼ cup of pecans toasted
- 2 tbsp crumbled feta cheese (optional)
- For the Dressing:
- 2 tbsp balsamic vinegar
- 1 tbsp olive oil
- 1 tsp honey or maple syrup
- Salt and pepper to taste

Instructions:

1. Add spinach, cut strawberries, and toasted nuts in a large mixing bowl.
2. Mix the balsamic vinegar, olive oil, honey, salt, and pepper in a small bowl until thoroughly blended.
3. Drizzle the dressing over the salad and gently mix to combine.
4. If desired, top with crumbled feta cheese for extra taste.
5. Serve immediately as a fresh, colorful salad.

Nutrition Information (per serving):

Calories: 160 Protein: 3g Carbohydrates: 14g Fat: 11g Fiber: 4g Sugar: 8g

Mediterranean Couscous Salad with Feta

Prep Time: 10 minutes

Cook Time: 10 minutes

Serving: 4

Ingredients:

- 1 cup of couscous
- 1 cup of water or vegetable broth
- ½ cup of cherry tomatoes, halved
- ½ cup of cucumber, diced
- ¼ cup of Kalamata olives, sliced
- ¼ cup of crumbled feta cheese
- 2 tbsp fresh parsley, chopped
- 1 tbsp fresh mint, chopped (optional)
- For the Dressing:
- 2 tbsp olive oil
- 2 tbsp fresh lemon juice
- 1 tsp Dijon mustard
- Salt and pepper to taste

Instructions:

1. Heat the water or vegetable broth in a medium saucepan until it boils. Remove from heat, toss in the couscous, cover, and set aside for 5 minutes. Fluff with a fork and let cool somewhat.
2. In a large bowl, mix the couscous, cherry tomatoes, cucumber, Kalamata olives, crumbled feta, parsley, and mint (if using).
3. Combine the olive oil, lemon juice, Dijon mustard, salt, and pepper in a small mixing bowl.
4. Pour the dressing over the couscous salad and toss to coat.
5. Serve chilled.

Nutrition Information (per serving):

Calories: 200 Protein: 6g Carbohydrates: 26g Fat: 9g Fiber: 3g Sugar: 2g

Broccoli and Almond Salad with a Honey Dressing

Prep Time: 10 minutes

Cook Time: N/A

Serving: 4

Ingredients:

- 4 cups of broccoli florets, chopped
- ¼ cup of sliced almonds toasted
- ¼ cup of dried cranberries (optional)
- ¼ small red onion, finely chopped
- For the Honey Dressing:
- 2 tbsp olive oil
- 1 tbsp honey
- 1 tbsp apple cider vinegar
- 1 tsp Dijon mustard
- Salt and pepper to taste

Instructions:

1. In a large mixing bowl, combine the broccoli, roasted almonds, dried cranberries (if using), and diced red onion.
2. Mix the olive oil, honey, apple cider vinegar, Dijon mustard, salt, and pepper in a small bowl.
3. Toss the broccoli mixture with the honey dressing until evenly coated.
4. Serve immediately.

Nutrition Information (per serving):

Calories: 150 Protein: 4g Carbohydrates: 13g Fat: 10g Fiber: 3g Sugar: 7g

Roasted Carrots with Thyme and Olive Oil

Prep Time: 5 minutes

Cook Time: 25 minutes

Serving: 4

Ingredients:

- 1 lb carrots, peeled and cut into sticks
- 2 tbsp olive oil
- 1 tsp fresh thyme leaves
- Salt and pepper to taste

Instructions:

1. Preheat the oven to 400 degrees Fahrenheit (200 degrees Celsius) and line a baking sheet with parchment paper.
2. Combine the carrot sticks, olive oil, thyme, salt, and pepper in a large mixing bowl.
3. Place the carrots in a single layer on the prepared baking sheet.
4. Roast the carrots for 20-25 minutes, rotating halfway through, until soft and gently caramelized.
5. Remove from the oven and serve warm as a tasty side dish.

Nutrition Information (per serving):

Calories: 120 Protein: 1g Carbohydrates: 11g Fat: 7g Fiber: 4g Sugar: 6g

Avocado and Tomato Salad with Balsamic Drizzle

Prep Time: 10 minutes

Cook Time: N/A

Serving: 2

Ingredients:

- 1 ripe avocado, diced
- 1 cup of cherry tomatoes, halved
- ¼ small red onion, thinly sliced
- 2 tbsp fresh basil leaves, chopped (optional)
- 2 tbsp balsamic vinegar
- 1 tbsp olive oil
- Salt and pepper to taste

Instructions:

1. In a mixing bowl, carefully combine the chopped avocado, cherry tomatoes, red onion, and basil (if using).
2. Combine the balsamic vinegar, olive oil, salt, and pepper in a small bowl.
3. Drizzle the balsamic mixture over the tomato and avocado salad.
4. Toss lightly to coat, then serve immediately.

Nutrition Information (per serving):

Calories: 180 Protein: 2g Carbohydrates: 12g Fat: 15g Fiber: 6g Sugar: 5g

Cauliflower Mash with Garlic and Olive Oil

Prep Time: 10 minutes

Cook Time: 15 minutes

Serving: 4

Ingredients:

- 1 large head of cauliflower, cut into florets
- 2 garlic cloves, minced
- 2 tbsp olive oil
- ¼ cup of unsweetened almond milk
- Salt and pepper to taste
- Fresh parsley, chopped (for garnish, optional)

Instructions:

1. Heat a large saucepan of water to a boil. Cook the cauliflower florets for 10-12 minutes or until soft.
2. Drain the cauliflower and add it to a food processor.
3. Mix the minced garlic, olive oil, almond milk, salt, and pepper with the cauliflower. Blend until smooth and creamy.
4. Taste and adjust the seasoning as required.
5. Serve warm as a nutritious alternative to mashed potatoes, garnished with chopped parsley as desired.

Nutrition Information (per serving):

Calories: 90 Protein: 3g Carbohydrates: 9g Fat: 6g Fiber: 3g Sugar: 2g

Lentil Salad with Feta and Herbs

Prep Time: 10 minutes

Cook Time: 20 minutes

Serving: 4

Ingredients:

- 1 cup of dried lentils, rinsed and drained
- 2 cups of water or vegetable broth
- ½ cup of crumbled feta cheese
- 1 small cucumber, diced
- 1 small red onion, finely chopped
- 2 tbsp fresh parsley, chopped
- 1 tbsp fresh mint, chopped (optional)
- For the Dressing:
- 2 tbsp olive oil
- 2 tbsp fresh lemon juice
- 1 tsp Dijon mustard
- Salt and pepper to taste

Instructions:

1. Heat the water or vegetable broth in a medium saucepan until it boils. Add the lentils, decrease the heat to low, cover, and cook for 20 minutes or until soft but not mushy. Drain the excess liquid and let the lentils cool somewhat.
2. In a large mixing bowl, combine the cooked lentils, crumbled feta, sliced cucumber, minced red onion, parsley, and mint (if desired).
3. Combine the olive oil, lemon juice, Dijon mustard, salt, and pepper in a small mixing bowl.
4. Pour the dressing over the lentils and toss to coat evenly.
5. Serve chilled or at room temperature for a refreshing and nutritional salad.

Nutrition Information (per serving):

Calories: 250 Protein: 12g Carbohydrates: 30g Fat: 10g Fiber: 8g Sugar: 3g

Grilled Zucchini with Lemon and Parmesan

Prep Time: 5 minutes

Cook Time: 10 minutes

Serving: 2

Ingredients:

- 2 medium zucchinis, sliced lengthwise into ¼-inch thick strips
- 1 tbsp olive oil
- Zest of 1 lemon
- 2 tbsp grated Parmesan cheese
- Salt and pepper to taste
- Fresh parsley, chopped (for garnish, optional)

Instructions:

1. Preheat the grill or grill pan to medium-high heat.
2. Brush olive oil onto the zucchini slices and season with salt and pepper.
3. Grill the zucchini on each side for 3-4 minutes until tender and faintly browned.
4. Place the grilled zucchini on a serving platter and garnish with lemon zest and grated Parmesan cheese.
5. Garnish with fresh parsley if preferred, and serve immediately.

Nutrition Information (per serving):

Calories: 120 Protein: 4g Carbohydrates: 6g Fat: 9g Fiber: 2g Sugar: 3g

DESSERTS

Coconut Chia Pudding with Fresh Mango

Prep Time: 10 minutes

Chilling time: 4 hours

Serving: 2

Ingredients:

- 1 cup of unsweetened coconut milk
- 3 tbsp chia seeds
- 1 tbsp honey or maple syrup (optional)
- ½ tsp vanilla extract
- 1 ripe mango, peeled and diced

Instructions:

1. Add coconut milk, chia seeds, honey (if using), and vanilla essence in a mixing bowl or container. Stir thoroughly to ensure that the chia seeds are uniformly dispersed.
2. Cover and chill for at least 4 hours, preferably overnight, to allow the chia seeds to absorb the liquid and thicken into a pudding-like texture.
3. When ready to serve, whisk the chia pudding to blend thoroughly.
4. Garnish with fresh diced mango and serve chilled.

Nutrition Information (per serving):

Calories: 200 Protein: 3g Carbohydrates: 22g Fat: 11g Fiber: 7g Sugar: 15g

Baked Apple with Cinnamon and Walnuts

Prep Time: 5 minutes

Cook Time: 20 minutes

Serving: 2

Ingredients:

- 2 medium apples, cored
- 2 tbsp chopped walnuts
- 1 tsp ground cinnamon
- 1 tbsp honey or maple syrup (optional)
- 1 tbsp raisins (optional)

Instructions:

1. Preheat the oven to 350° Fahrenheit (175° Celsius).
2. Place the cored apples onto a small baking dish.
3. In a small bowl, combine the chopped walnuts, cinnamon, and honey (if using). If desired, stir in the raisins.
4. Fill the middle of each apple with walnut mixture.
5. Bake the apples for 20 minutes or until they are soft. Serve warm as a warming and nutritious dessert.

Nutrition Information (per serving):

Calories: 160 Protein: 2g Carbohydrates: 28g Fat: 6g Fiber: 5g Sugar: 22g

Dark Chocolate Avocado Mousse

Prep Time: 10 minutes

Cook Time: N/A

Serving: 2

Ingredients:

- 1 ripe avocado
- 3 tbsp unsweetened cocoa powder
- 2 tbsp honey or maple syrup
- 1 tsp vanilla extract
- 2 tbsp almond milk
- Pinch of sea salt
- Fresh berries or grated dark chocolate

Instructions:

1. Mix avocado, cocoa powder, honey or maple syrup, vanilla extract, almond milk, and a sprinkling of sea salt in a blender or food processor.
2. Blend until smooth and creamy, scraping down the sides as necessary.
3. Taste and adjust the sweetness to your liking.
4. Spoon the mousse into serving dishes and chill for 30 minutes.
5. Garnish with fresh berries or grated dark chocolate before serving.

Nutrition Information (per serving):

Calories: 220 Protein: 3g Carbohydrates: 26g Fat: 14g Fiber: 7g Sugar: 18g

Blueberry-Almond Crumble

Prep Time: 10 minutes

Cook Time: 25 minutes

Serving: 4

Ingredients:

- For the Filling:
- 2 cups of fresh or frozen blueberries
- 1 tbsp honey or maple syrup
- 1 tbsp lemon juice
- 1 tsp vanilla extract
- For the Crumble Topping:
- ½ cup of almond flour
- ¼ cup of rolled oats (optional for texture)
- ¼ cup of sliced almonds
- 2 tbsp coconut oil (or butter), melted
- 1 tbsp honey or maple syrup
- ½ tsp ground cinnamon
- Pinch of sea salt

Instructions:

1. Preheat the oven to 350° Fahrenheit (175° Celsius).
2. Combine the blueberries, honey, maple syrup, lemon juice, and vanilla essence in a medium mixing bowl. Mix thoroughly and evenly distribute the blueberry mixture in a baking dish.
3. In a separate mixing bowl, combine the almond flour, rolled oats (if using), sliced almonds, melted coconut oil, honey or maple syrup, cinnamon, and salt until crumbly.
4. Sprinkle the crumble topping evenly over the blueberry mixture.
5. Bake for 20-25 minutes until the top is golden brown and the blueberries are bubbling.
6. Remove from the oven and allow to cool slightly before serving.

Nutrition Information (per serving):

Calories: 220 Protein: 4g Carbohydrates: 26g Fat: 12g Fiber: 5g Sugar: 15g

Baked Pears with Honey and Almonds

Prep Time: 5 minutes

Cook Time: 20 minutes

Serving: 2

Ingredients:

- 2 ripe pears, halved and cored
- 2 tbsp honey
- ¼ tsp ground cinnamon
- 2 tbsp sliced almonds
- 1 tbsp coconut oil (or butter), melted

Instructions:

1. Preheat the oven to 350° Fahrenheit (175° Celsius).
2. Place the cut side of the pear halves up on a baking tray. Drizzle the pears with honey and melted coconut oil, then finish with cinnamon.
3. Spread the sliced almonds on top of the pears.
4. Bake the pears for 15-20 minutes or until soft. Serve warm for an easy and nutritious dessert.

Nutrition Information (per serving):

Calories: 180 Protein: 2g Carbohydrates: 31g Fat: 7g Fiber: 5g Sugar: 25g

Chia Seed Pudding with Coconut and Berries

Prep Time: 5 minutes

Chilling time: 4 hours (or overnight)

Serving: 2

Ingredients:

- 1 cup of unsweetened coconut milk
- 3 tbsp chia seeds
- 1 tbsp honey or maple syrup (optional)
- ½ tsp vanilla extract
- ¼ cup of shredded unsweetened coconut
- ½ cup of fresh mixed berries (blueberries, raspberries, or strawberries)

Instructions:

1. In a bowl or container, combine the coconut milk, chia seeds, honey (if using), and vanilla essence. Stir thoroughly to ensure that the chia seeds are uniformly dispersed.
2. Cover and chill for at least 4 hours, preferably overnight, to allow the chia seeds to absorb the liquid and develop a pudding-like texture.
3. Once the chia pudding has set, mix it and divide it into serving dishes.
4. Garnish with shredded coconut and fresh mixed berries.
5. Serve chilled for a tasty and nutritious snack or dessert.

Nutrition Information (per serving):

Calories: 220 Protein: 4g Carbohydrates: 20g Fat: 15g Fiber: 9g Sugar: 10g

Banana Oat Cookies with Dark Chocolate Chips

Prep Time: 10 minutes

Cook Time: 15 minutes

Serving: 12 cookies

Ingredients:

- 2 ripe bananas, mashed
- 1 ½ cups of rolled oats
- ¼ cup of almond butter (or any nut butter)
- 2 tbsp honey or maple syrup (optional)
- ¼ tsp ground cinnamon
- ¼ cup of dark chocolate chips
- 1 tsp vanilla extract
- Pinch of salt

Instructions:

1. Preheat the oven to 350°F/175°C and line a baking sheet with parchment paper.
2. In a large bowl, combine the mashed bananas, almond butter, honey (if using), vanilla essence, and a sprinkle of salt until thoroughly blended.
3. Combine the rolled oats, cinnamon, and dark chocolate chips.
4. Drop spoonful of cookie dough onto the prepared baking sheet, flattening them slightly with the back of a spoon.
5. Bake for 12 to 15 minutes or until the cookies are gently brown and firm.
6. Allow the cookies to cool on the baking sheet for a few minutes before moving them to a wire rack to finish cooling.

Nutrition Information (per cookie):

Calories: 110 Protein: 3g Carbohydrates: 18g Fat: 4g Fiber: 3g Sugar: 7g

Almond Flour Brownies with Walnuts

Prep Time: 10 minutes

Cook Time: 25 minutes

Serving: 9 squares

Ingredients:

- 1 cup of almond flour
- ¼ cup of unsweetened cocoa powder
- ¼ tsp baking soda
- ¼ tsp salt
- ¼ cup of coconut oil, melted
- ¼ cup of honey or maple syrup
- 2 large eggs
- 1 tsp vanilla extract
- ½ cup of dark chocolate chips
- ¼ cup of chopped walnuts

Instructions:

1. Preheat the oven to 350°F (175°C) and line an 8-by-8-inch baking sheet with parchment paper.
2. Combine the almond flour, cocoa powder, baking soda, and salt in a larger bowl.
3. Combine the melted coconut oil, honey or maple syrup, eggs, and vanilla extract in a separate bowl. Whisk until creamy.
4. Combine the wet and dry ingredients and whisk until completely combined.
5. Fold in the dark chocolate chips and chopped walnuts. Pour the batter into the prepared baking pan and distribute evenly.
6. Bake for 20 to 25 minutes or until a toothpick inserted in the middle comes out clean.
7. Allow the brownies to cool fully in their pan before cutting them into squares.

Nutrition Information (per square):

Calories: 180 Protein: 4g Carbohydrates: 14g Fat: 12g Fiber: 3g Sugar: 10g

Pumpkin Spice Energy Balls

Prep Time: 10 minutes

Chilling time: 30 minutes

Serving: 12 energy balls

Ingredients:

- 1 cup of rolled oats
- ¼ cup of almond butter (or any nut butter)
- ¼ cup of pumpkin puree
- 2 tbsp honey or maple syrup
- 1 tsp vanilla extract
- 1 tsp pumpkin pie spice
- 2 tbsp chia seeds (optional)
- ¼ cup of dark chocolate chips (optional)

Instructions:

1. Add rolled oats, almond butter, pumpkin puree, honey or maple syrup, vanilla essence, and pumpkin pie spice in a large mixing bowl.
2. Stir in the chia seeds and dark chocolate chips, if using, until well combined.
3. Roll the mixture into tiny balls (approximately 1 tbsp each) and place on a baking sheet lined with parchment paper.
4. Refrigerate the energy balls for at least 30 minutes until firm.
5. Refrigerate in an airtight container for up to a week.

Nutrition Information (per energy ball):

Calories: 90 Protein: 2g Carbohydrates: 12g Fat: 4g Fiber: 2g Sugar: 6g

21 DAYS MEAL PLAN

Day	Breakfast	Lunch	Dinner	Snacks
01	Quinoa Porridge with Berries and Almonds	Grilled Salmon Salad with Avocado and Lemon Dressing	Baked Salmon with Roasted Brussels Sprouts	Roasted Chickpeas with Paprika
02	Spinach and Mushroom Scramble with Avocado	Quinoa and Roasted Vegetable Bowl	Grilled Chicken Breast with Sweet Potato Mash	Veggie Sticks with Hummus
03	Chia Seed Pudding with Blueberries	Lentil and Spinach Soup	Turmeric-Ginger Chicken Stir-Fry with Vegetables	Apple Slices with Almond Butter and Cinnamon
04	Oatmeal with Walnuts and Flaxseeds	Chickpea and Cucumber Salad with Tahini Dressing	Lentil and Vegetable Shepherd's Pie	Greek Yogurt with Walnuts and Honey
05	Sweet Potato and Kale Hash	Turkey and Veggie Lettuce Wraps	Baked Cod with Lemon and Garlic Green Beans	Kale Chips with Nutritional Yeast
06	Veggie-Packed Omelet with Herbs	Veggie-Loaded Quinoa Stuffed Peppers	Grilled Tofu and Veggie Skewers with Brown Rice	Sweet Potato Chips with Guacamole
07	Coconut Yogurt Parfait with Mixed Berries	Zucchini Noodles with Pesto and Grilled Chicken	Chickpea and Spinach Curry with Cauliflower Rice	Edamame with Sea Salt and Lemon
08	Almond Butter Toast with Banana and Hemp Seeds	Wild Rice and Black Bean Salad with Citrus Dressing	Turkey Meatballs with Zucchini Noodles and Tomato Sauce	Almond-Coconut Energy Bites
09	Avocado and Tomato Breakfast Sandwich on Whole Grain Bread	Mediterranean Chickpea and Farro Salad	Moroccan-Spiced Vegetable Tagine with Couscous	Baked Zucchini Fries with Spicy Yogurt Dip
10	Turmeric-Spiced Oatmeal with Chia Seeds	Spinach and Quinoa Wrap with Hummus	Baked Tilapia with Sautéed Spinach and Mushrooms	Roasted Beet Chips with Tahini Dip
11	Buckwheat Pancakes with Fresh Berries	Grilled Chicken and Mango Salad with Cilantro Lime Dressing	Black Bean and Sweet Potato Enchiladas	Cucumber and Radish Salad with Lemon Vinaigrette
12	Poached Eggs on a Bed of Sautéed Greens	Roasted Beet and Feta Salad with Walnuts	Sautéed Shrimp with Quinoa and Broccoli	Veggie Sticks with Hummus
13	Millet Porridge with Dried Fruit and Pumpkin Seeds	Brown Rice Sushi Rolls with Avocado and Cucumber	Roasted Turkey Breast with Mashed Cauliflower	Roasted Chickpeas with Paprika
14	Sweet Potato Breakfast Bowl with Spinach and Tahini	Mediterranean Couscous Salad with Feta	Tempeh Stir-Fry with Broccoli and Peppers	Baked Carrot Fries with Curry Dip

15	Banana and Almond Smoothie Bowl	Wild Rice Pilaf with Cranberries and Almonds	Roasted Sweet Potatoes with Cinnamon and Olive Oil	Grilled Eggplant with Chickpea Salad
16	Quinoa Porridge with Berries and Almonds	Baked Cod with Lemon and Garlic Green Beans	Grilled Chicken Breast with Sweet Potato Mash	Edamame with Sea Salt and Lemon
17	Coconut Yogurt Parfait with Mixed Berries	Lentil and Spinach Soup	Chickpea and Spinach Curry with Cauliflower Rice	Blueberry-Almond Crumble
18	Spinach and Mushroom Scramble with Avocado	Quinoa and Roasted Vegetable Bowl	Turmeric-Ginger Chicken Stir-Fry with Vegetables	Apple Slices with Almond Butter and Cinnamon
19	Oatmeal with Walnuts and Flaxseeds	Chickpea and Cucumber Salad with Tahini Dressing	Lentil and Vegetable Shepherd's Pie	Kale Chips with Nutritional Yeast
20	Sweet Potato and Kale Hash	Turkey and Veggie Lettuce Wraps	Grilled Tofu and Veggie Skewers with Brown Rice	Sweet Potato Chips with Guacamole
21	Veggie-Packed Omelet with Herbs	Zucchini Noodles with Pesto and Grilled Chicken	Moroccan-Spiced Vegetable Tagine with Couscous	Greek Yogurt with Walnuts and Honey

Printed in Great Britain
by Amazon